Neuropharmacology and Behavior

V. G. Longo

Istituto Superiore di Sanità
Rome

with a Foreword by
James L. McGaugh
University of California
Irvine

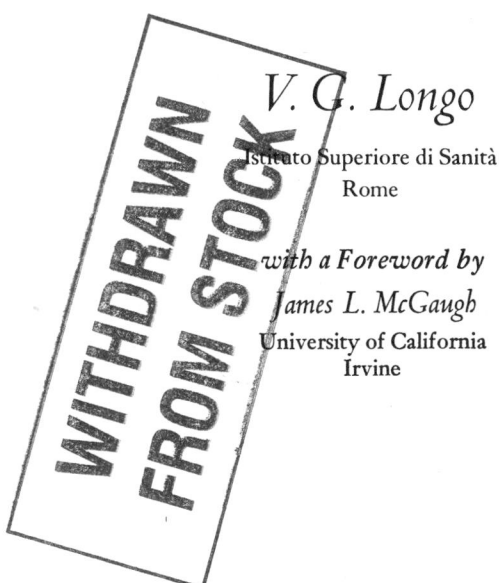

W. H. Freeman and Company
San Francisco

Printed in the United States of America

International Standard Book Number: 0-7167-0828-0 (cloth)
0-7167-0827-2 (paper)

Library of Congress Catalog Card Number: 72-75588

1 2 3 4 5 6 7 8 9

To my wife

Contents

Foreword

Man has known for many centuries that his behavior and experience are profoundly influenced by drugs. It is only in recent years that we have achieved systematic understanding of the nature and bases of drug influences on behavior. Such understanding is essential for the development of rational chemical therapies for mental disorders as well as for dealing with the persistent and growing problem of drug abuse.

Developments in neuropsychopharmacology have occurred extremely rapidly in the past two decades. In this timely book Professor Longo has provided a careful, selective, and coherent summary of current knowledge of the history, use, therapeutic effectiveness, and neurobiological effects of some of the drugs which significantly alter behavior and experience.

JAMES L. MCGAUGH

Preface

This book should not be considered as an attempt to describe and explain, all inclusively, the techniques, results, and theories related to neuropharmacology. When writing the manuscript, I was profoundly biased by my own interests, and the present work is, in a sense, autobiographical, being an extension and elaboration of the several investigations I have carried out in the fields of neuropharmacology and behavior. I am, in fact, one of the people who, upon entering medical research when neuropharmacology was in its infancy, became interested in it and continued in the field to the present day; indeed, it has been very rewarding, in the course of the preparation of this book, to recall and record many of the remarkable developments that have occurred during these years and in which I participated.

Altogether, the following material is presented from the viewpoint of a practicing scientist who has learned the hard way; it seems to me that this puts me in a good position to inform the reader in a straightforward fashion of techniques pertinent to the study of centrally acting agents, of results obtained in animals and man, and of theories elaborated to explain the mechanism of action of these agents.

As a difficult situation prevailed at the Istituto di Sanità during the last few years, the writing of this book provided consolation and optimism.

If the reader finds the English text clear and easy to follow, this is due in a large part to the assistance of Professor A. G. Karczmar and of Dr. W. De Maio, who spent hours correcting my mistakes and putting the manuscript in good form. I also thank those authors and publishers who granted the permission for the use of certain materials.

Finally, I should like to acknowledge the suggestions, the help, and the sympathy received from my wife, to whom this book is dedicated.

V. G. LONGO

May, 1972

Neuropharmacology
and Behavior

Chemotherapy
of Mental Diseases

The following chapters will deal with a group of drugs—namely, antipsychotics, antidepressives, and tranquilizers—whose development represents a great advance in the treatment of mental diseases.

Before the early 1950s, the armamentarium of drugs available for the treatment of psychotic patients was very limited, and the efficacy and mode of action of the drugs were such that few patients derived a marked benefit from them. Drugs were of secondary importance relative to other forms of therapy, such as shock therapy and psychotherapy. Generally, before the early 1950s patients had to be permanently hospitalized.

The advent of what is called the chemotherapy of mental diseases goes back to the years 1952–1953. At that time, chlorpromazine was introduced in the treatment of various psychiatric conditions; this was followed by the introduction of reserpine, which had a similar application, and of meprobamate (Miltown) which was used for the relief of anxiety (Délay and Deniker, 1961). The first observations dealing with the usefulness of these drugs in neuropsychiatric patients occurred in clinics. Many clinical reports dealing with the chemotherapy of mental diseases appeared almost simultaneously. This may seem astonishing; however, a more careful look at the situation reveals a rich background of pharmacological and clinical research, from which the discovery of these drugs stemmed directly and as a matter of course. Although the major part of the pharmacological and clinical research preceding 1952–1953 was not aimed directly at mental diseases, the literature of this time indicated that the attention of investigators was focusing more and more on the actions of various drugs on the central nervous system. Their observations concerned: the soporific effect of certain antihistaminics (such as promethazine); the antiemetic and anti-motion-sickness effect of other antihistaminics (diphenhydramine); the applications of synthetic atropinics and spasmolytics (caramiphen, diethazine) in the therapy of parkinsonism; the sedative actions of the muscle-relaxant mephenesin; the drowsiness and the depressive syndrome observed in the course of treatment of hypertensive patients with rauwolfia extracts. One can readily see how the groundwork was laid for more specific applications of drugs of this type in the therapy of mental diseases.

The upsurge of research that followed the first reports of the positive therapeutic effects of the new drugs was characterized by a close cooperation between pharmacologists and clinicians; the advent of this collaboration constitutes the birth of neuropsychopharmacology as a discipline. The successive introduction in the clinic of new products led to rapid progress and the firm establishment of this discipline; the armamentarium of drugs for the treatment of mental diseases became gradually richer both qualitatively and quantitatively. In 1955, Jacobsen described the "ataraxic" effect of benactyzine, which for a limited time was employed in the treatment of neurosis. In 1957, two drug prototypes were introduced almost simultaneously for the therapy of depressive syndromes: iproniazid, an inhibitor of monoamine oxidase (Loomer et al., 1957), and imipramine, a tricyclic drug that chemically, but not clinically, resembled chlorpromazine. Chlorpromazine served as a model for synthesis of hundreds of related products, as every pharmaceutical company competed for the development of an antipsychotic. Similarly, with regard to rauwolfia, new alkaloids were isolated, and the molecule of reserpine itself was manipulated. A more original departure occurred with the development of butyrophenones, drugs with an antipsychotic profile, among which the most effective currently available antipsychotic drugs can be found. Finally, in the field of anti-anxiety agents, other substances became available; in particular, the benzodiazepine derivatives proved more potent than meprobamate in the treatment of anxiety.

Following this period of intense activity, which lasted some ten years, there ensued a phase of evaluation, during which many substances were considered more critically and vanished from the clinical scene. Countless congresses, symposia, and round tables followed one another, with the purpose of classifying the various effects of the new drugs and of comparing the effects in man with the experimental animal data. New interdisciplinary organizations and publications contributed to the dissemination of pertinent information.

The task of classifying and characterizing the new products proved arduous, as is demonstrated by the very numerous attempts to devise a comprehensive system of classification. One of the most ingenious schemes of pharmacological and clinical properties of the various products was proposed by Jacobsen (1959) in one of the early reviews on the subject (Figure 1.1). This complicated scheme illustrates very well the problems associated with the overlap and multiplicity of the properties in question, as well as the difficulty of establishing clear-cut divisions.

In the present review, these drugs have been subdivided into three groups: the antipsychotics, the antidepressants, and the tranquilizers. The antipsychotics, which are also called *neuroleptics* or *major tranquilizers*, comprise the phenothiazines, reserpine and its analogs, and the butyrophenones. The tranquilizers, referred to sometimes as *minor tranquilizers, anxiolytics* or *anti-anxiety agents*, include meprobamate and its analogs and the benzodiazepines. Finally, the antidepressants consist of two subgroups: on the one hand the antidepressants that are inhibitors of monoamine oxidase (MAO), and on the other the so-called tricyclic antidepressants that are not MAO inhibitors.

THE CLINICAL APPLICATION

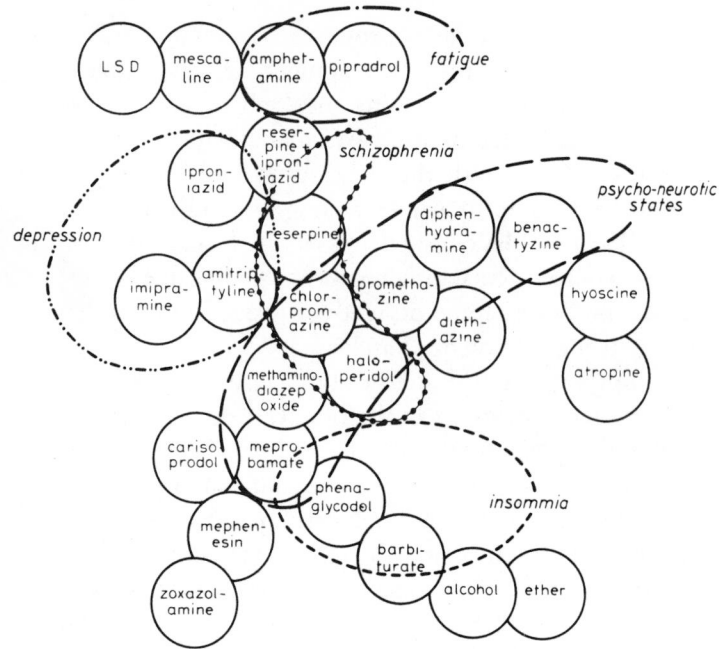

PSYCHOTROPIC DRUGS AND THEIR EFFECTS

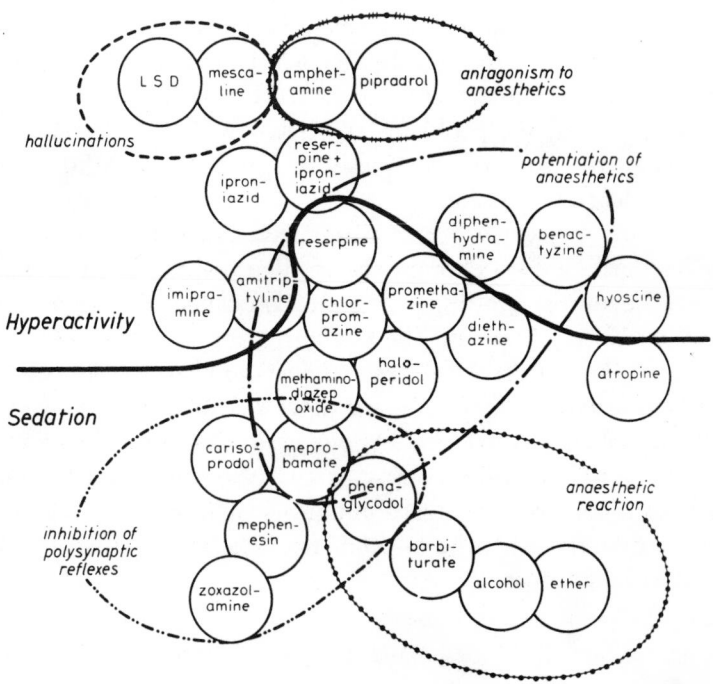

AUTONOMIC EFFECTS

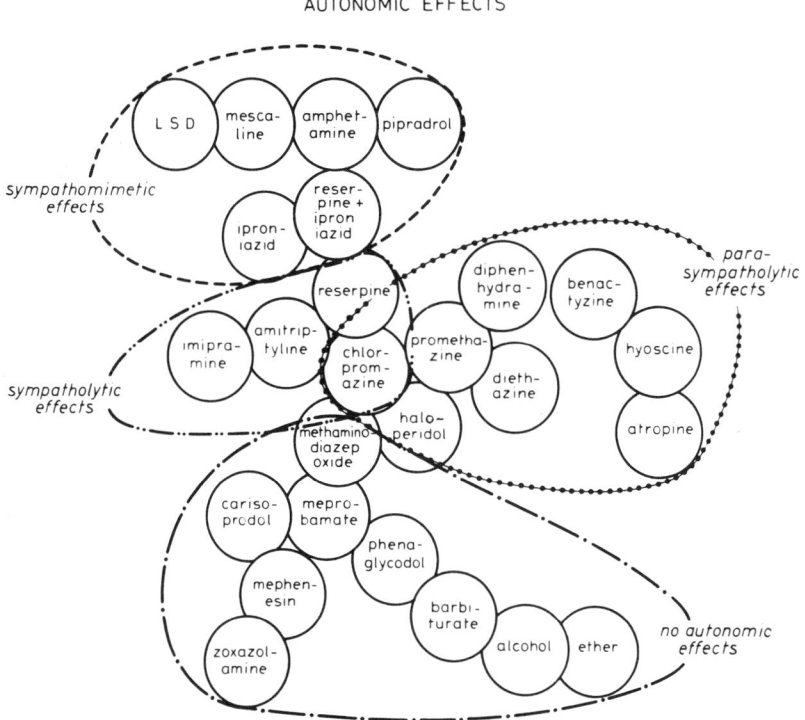

Figure 1.1
These diagrams are redrawn from papers published by Jacobsen in 1959 and 1963. On the basis of the data available at that time, some psychotropic drugs are grouped according to various types of action.

For the reasons already given, it is difficult to devise an overall description of properties that will hold for *all* the drugs in a particular group; however, the following general scheme was prepared to help the reader attain an overview of the field.

1. Antipsychotic, or neuroleptic, drugs are characterized by: (*a*) induction of tranquilization and mental relaxation; (*b*) high efficacy in obtunding the overt symptoms of acute and chronic psychotic patients; (*c*) causation of reversible extrapyramidal side effects; (*d*) lack of habituation and dependence.
2. Depression is often a self-limiting illness. It is therefore difficult to evaluate the effect of antidepressives on "melancholic" individuals. The following, however, may be stated. The tricyclic

antidepressants, such as imipramine, are characterized by: (*a*) effectiveness in psychotic depression; (*b*) delayed appearance of beneficial effects (up to three weeks); (*c*) side effects mainly due to their atropine-like action. The antidepressants of the MAO-inhibitor type: (*a*) are effective with respect to neurotic or hysterical depression; (*b*) exhibit a more rapid onset of effect; (*c*) have important and dangerous side effects: they potentiate the effects of many drugs, therefore hindering combined treatment; they produce hypotension, constipation, and dysuria; they have a marked hepato-toxicity. Despite all this, the general consensus is that there is a definite place in psychiatry for the use of these drugs.

3. The tranquilizers exhibit the following properties: (*a*) they induce tranquilization and mental relaxation; (*b*) they are effective in nervous tension, common neurotic syndromes, psychosomatic disorders; (*c*) physical dependence does occur sometimes.

References

Délay, J., and Deniker, P. *Méthodes Chimiothérapeutiques en Psychiatrie*, Masson, Paris, 1961.

Jacobsen, E. *Bull. World Health Organ.* 21:411, 1959.

Jacobsen, E. *Int. J. Neuropsychiat.* 4:241, 1963.

Loomer, H. P., et al. *Psychiatric. Res. Rep.* 8:129, 1957.

CHAPTER 1

Antipsychotic Drugs

CHLORPROMAZINE AND THE RELATED PHENOTHIAZINES

In the course of the Second World War, chemists of the French Rhône-Poulenc Company embarked upon synthesis of a series of derivatives of phenothiazine, a nucleus that was already known and had been worked with for quite a long time. Some of the compounds thus obtained exhibited a combination of antihistaminic, atropinic, and ganglioplegic properties. In 1946 it was reported that certain phenothiazine derivatives were successful in the therapy of parkinsonism (diethazine) and of allergic syndromes (promethazine). Although the work with these and related agents produced evidence of their sedative action, the key observation was made in 1952 by

Laborit et al. These researchers used a Rhône-Poulenc synthetic—developed a few years earlier as "RP 4560" and subsequently called chlorpromazine (CPZ)—as an ingredient of the *cocktail lytique,* employed for the potentiation of anesthesia and for the induction of "artificial hibernation." Their conceptualization was based not so much on the central effects of the drug, as on the atropinic, adrenolytic, antihistaminic and ganglioplegic effects, as demonstrated in the laboratory (Courvoisier et al., 1953). But Laborit et al. (1952) stressed the psychic effect of the drug, which at intravenous doses of 50–100 mg exhibited a peculiar sedative action, without loss of consciousness or alteration in mentation. We owe to Délay and his school a systematic study of CPZ in the treatment of mental diseases (see Délay and Deniker, 1961). In their first reports, in 1952, these authors gave chlorpromazine its name, describing in detail (*a*) the psychomotor depression that followed its administration and (*b*) its therapeutic action upon several psychoses. Subsequent investigations in Europe, Canada, and the United States confirmed and extended the observations of the French psychiatrists. It is of interest in this respect to mention that the approval for marketing CPZ in the United States was given for its use as an antiemetic. In fact, the clinical studies carried out in other countries were not considered sufficient to prove its efficacy in the treatment of mental illnesses; only following a thorough, well-controlled study, did the drug receive official approval as an antipsychotic.

Thus, CPZ opened the era of chemotherapy of mental illness and within a short period of time triggered a series of studies on its derivatives and analogs. The various phenothiazine derivatives differ both quantitatively and qualitatively in the way they affect the central nervous system and the peripheral nervous system. Numerous phenothiazines were introduced into therapy, some being used for the same symptoms that the mother substance is used for and some being used for more specific symptoms. The phenothiazines are commonly divided into three groups, as shown in Figure 1.2. The first group includes the compounds in which a three-carbon aliphatic side chain originates at the nitrogen of the median nucleus, terminating with a dimethylamino group. These compounds have both sedative and antipsychotic effects; the principal representative of this class is CPZ. In the second group, the aliphatic side chain terminates with a piperidine nucleus; the compounds of

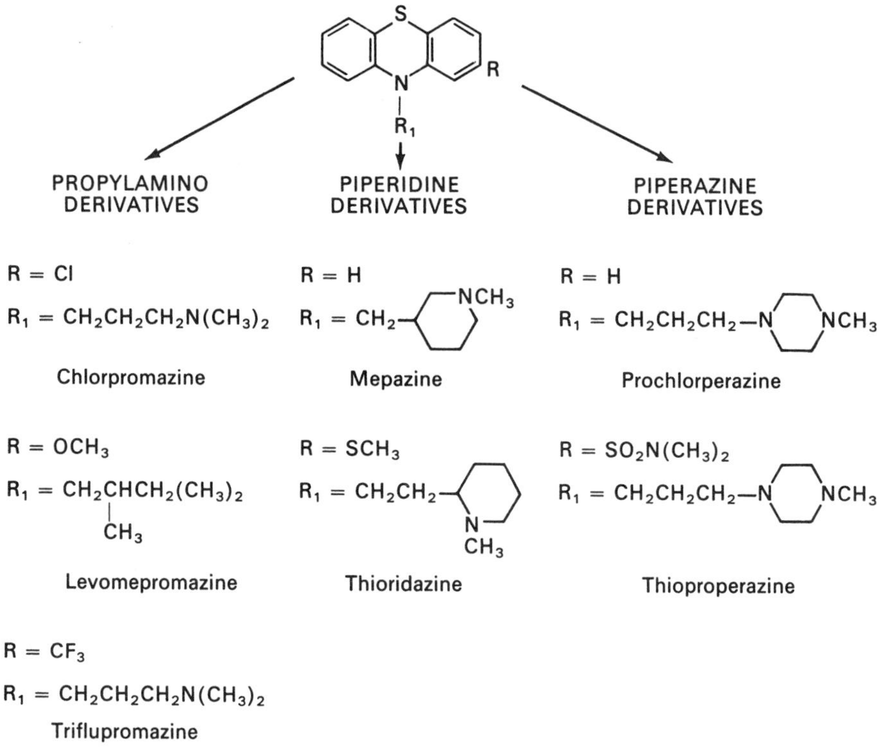

Figure 1.2
Here are a few examples of phenothiazine derivatives used in the clinic for their sedative and antipsychotic properties. The compounds are divided into three groups, according to the chemical nature of the side chain attached at the nitrogen of the median nucleus.

this group, such as mepazine and thioridazine, have sedative properties but are less effective as antipsychotics than compounds of the first group; however, they are less toxic and are easier to handle. A piperazine nucleus at the end of the side chain characterizes the drugs of the third group, the most potent antipsychotics, which exhibit a marked antiemetic effect; however, they are more toxic than the other compounds and cause intense side effects.

Several reviews of the vast amount of data on the phenothiazines are available, and the reader is referred to these publications for details (see Domino et al., 1968). Here, the effects of CPZ will be described, and the other phenothiazines will be compared to the mother drug as they apply.

Clinical Effects

According to Freyhan (1959), CPZ is "effective in the treatment of psychopathological states which have in common hypermotility, abnormal initiative, and increased affective tension." In practice the drug is widely used for symptomatic treatment of a number of psychiatric conditions, such as—

1. Schizophrenia: excitatory states, paranoid tension, stereotypic and bizarre activities, and destructive behavior.
2. Affective disorders: maniacal and hypomaniacal states.
3. Acute cerebral syndromes: states of intoxication, delirium, and hallucinations.
4. Chronic cerebral syndromes, particularly those that include agitation and confusion.

While it is true that, in general, the drug acts mainly on the symptoms, the results obtained in certain cases, as for instance in early schizophrenia, are so dramatic, and the return to normal is so complete and long-lasting, that one may ask if there is only a symptomatic amelioration or also a basic modification of the psychotic process. Putting aside these comments, which some may consider too optimistic, it cannot be denied that the introduction of this and other antipsychotic phenothiazines has brought many changes to psychiatric clinics. In the first place, the absolute number of patients has decreased (Figure 1.3). Prior to the advent of the phenothiazines, inpatients had little chance for return to a normal function within society; today, manic or schizophrenic patients treated with these neuroleptics may exhibit an amelioration that is so marked that it permits a successful return to society. Second, global treatment with neuroleptics of the patients in so-called "disturbed wards" markedly diminished the time spent in isolation, the number of broken windows, assaults on the staff and on other patients, and the use of restraints. Finally, the introduction of the neuroleptics has opened up the possibility of outpatient treatment of syndromes that previously could be dealt with only in a hospital.

Before we discuss in detail the effects of CPZ, it should be made clear that, although CPZ affects the normal individual (for instance, his psychomotor activity), we shall confine ourselves to its effects on the psychotic. A complete picture of the action of this

NUMBER OF RESIDENT PATIENTS IN STATE AND LOCAL
GOVERNMENT MENTAL HOSPITALS IN THE UNITED STATES
(based on USPHS Figures)
1946 -1967

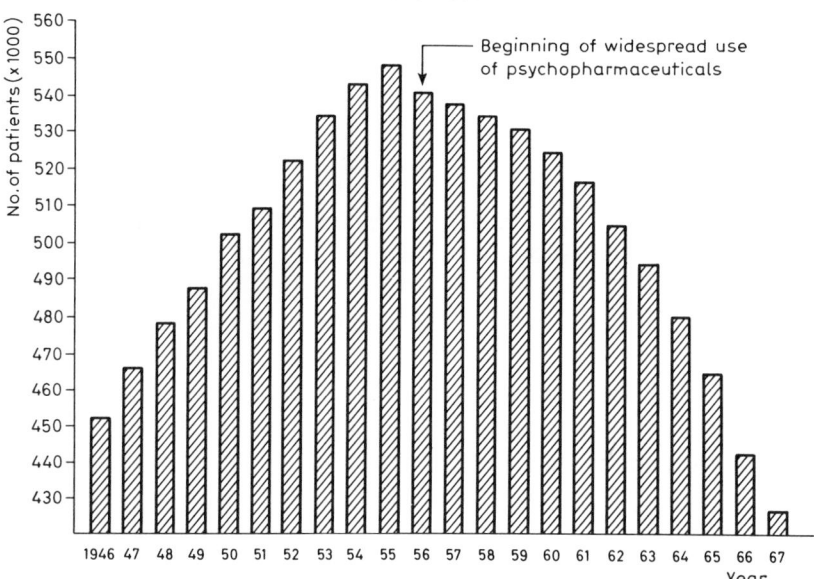

Figure 1.3
In 1967, the American College of Neuropsychopharmacology, jointly with the
NIMH, organized a meeting to discuss the progress of psychopharmacology in the
previous 10 years. In the course of his presidential address, Dr. N. S. Kline presented
a single slide showing the above graph, which reflects a dramatic change in the total
population of mental hospitals since the introduction of psychopharmaceuticals. A
further confirmation of the effectiveness of treatment is given by the two-fold increase in the live-discharge rate recorded since the introduction of these drugs
(modified, from Efron, 1968).

drug on a psychotic patient can be obtained only when a thorough,
objective analysis by those treating the patient is combined with a
subjective account by the patient himself. Thus, we shall consider
both points of view in the following discussion.

The affective tension that characterizes a psychotic is markedly
benefited by treatment. In psychotics this tension may be manifest
either in psychomotor agitation or in motor depression. In the former instance, the drug reduces excitation; in the latter, it restores
contact with the outside world, thus augmenting activity. The other

symptoms that respond to treatment are the delusions and hallucinations that frequently characterize schizophrenic episodes. The cessation of delusions and hallucinations is particularly dramatic when early cases of schizophrenia are treated. The patients' own subjective accounts of the changes permit us to appreciate the effectiveness of the drug; these accounts explain why the early reports on the clinical application of the drug were so enthusiastic.

The subjective effect of CPZ can be divided into two phases. The first phase occurs immediately: the patients report that they feel sleepy, tired, and weak. This weakness is experienced directly as a physical sensation: heaviness in the limbs, difficulties in walking, etc. Following this sedative effect, patients experience a second phase, in which paranoid and hallucinatory symptoms are reduced or ended.

Some examples (taken from Haase and Janssen, 1965) of verbatim reports from patients following neuroleptic treatment show a striking change in their outlooks.

> Patient 1: The medicine has done me good. A stimulating medicine wouldn't have helped get my thoughts in order. The excitement inside stops the thoughts from settling down, instead they keep coming into mind. Now, however, I am completely normal. Since coming here, I've grown calmer and at the same time the confused thoughts have disappeared. Also the idea of being persecuted. Nowadays I laugh about it. At home I always used to pep myself up with coffee and cigarettes so that I could read more intensely. I did this to such a pitch, that I started to get all confused. The medicine here has calmed me down, so naturally the confusion has disappeared.

> Patient 2: The tablets calm me down so that my nature doesn't come out. Everything is so unimportant to me, I couldn't care less where I am, here or somewhere else. I used to say I was a "Royal Charlady," but that was all madness. I only imagined it.

> Patient 3: I think the disconnected thoughts have disappeared because the brain has begun to work more quietly. I see now that the voices and thoughts that I have had were all imaginary. During my illness I had no energy. Now it's slowly coming back. I can only think that my energy was in some way "wrongly connected" and that was the cause of it.

The lowering of the psychoenergetic level, observed during the first phase of the drug's action, is observable also in normal individuals treated with phenothiazines; in fact, in these subjects, this is the only effect of the drug. It should be added in this context that a comparison in normal subjects of chlorpromazine and promethazine (an antihistaminic with no antipsychotic properties) revealed little difference between the effect of the two drugs (Hollister, 1968).

An important practical consideration is that CPZ induces in psychotics the effects described without impairing consciousness and judgment. Therefore, a patient, relieved of his anxiety and paranoia, becomes responsive to psychotherapy. It is during this period that he may learn that there are other ways to deal with his problems; through the assistance of a specialized staff he may make further progress. By contrast, drugs that were used before the advent of phenothiazines in the treatment of psychotic patients, such as bromides and barbiturates, had the disadvantage of causing withdrawal, somnolence, and, sometimes, sleep.

Although less spectacular, some positive results can sometimes be obtained with CPZ in chronic schizophrenics, particularly with regard to certain symptoms, such as negativism, lack of contact, and aggressive behavior. In some cases it makes possible the transfer of the patient from "custodial" to "active" wards.

In the control of overactive behavior and other symptoms of mania, the use of CPZ is limited to the treatment of acute episodes; the drug does not seem to prevent the course of the disease, during which spontaneous remissions alternate with periods of hypomania; in fact, the drug is contraindicated during the state of depression. CPZ has proved to be an useful tool in controlling acute reactions encountered in the course of toxic psychoses (such as those induced by LSD), delirium tremens, and posttraumatic states. Other phenothiazines (such as prochlorperazine, belonging to the piperazine group, Figure 1.2) are used as antiemetics, although CPZ is still widely employed, with dramatic results, in severe cases of emesis.

Because of its sedative properties, CPZ is also used in the treatment of neurosis, to control tension and anxiety; for these conditions the piperidine derivatives (see Figure 1.2) seem to be more indicated. (Today, however, the benzodiazepines are the treatment of choice for tension and anxiety.) The piperidine derivatives, at very low dose levels, show a feeble antidepressive action and are used, often in association with more specific drugs, in the treatment of psychotic depressions.

In general, CPZ is given orally. While in neuroses the drug is given in low doses (50–100 mg daily), a wide range of doses has been employed for the treatment of psychotic syndromes. In these cases, the dosage depends upon the individual response and can vary from 200 to 3600 mg daily. Usually, prolonged treatment is necessary. There is no evidence of tolerance; in the most favorable cases, the sedative effect diminishes while the antipsychotic effect remains unchanged. With most patients extrapyramidal side effects appear. In fact, it has been theorized that, in order to obtain a therapeutic action, the induction of these effects is a prerequisite. Three types of extrapyramidal side effects have been described: dystonic-dyskinetic crises, akathisia and tasikinesia, and the parkinsonian syndrome.

The dystonic crisis is observed particularly with phenothiazines of the piperazine group, and it usually occurs during the first days of treatment. The episodes have a sudden onset and a dramatic course: patients show facial grimacing, oculogyric crisis, torticollis, and sometimes opisthotonos. These attacks are often frightening and can be mistaken for tetanus or epileptic fits. Various interpretations have been presented to explain them—for instance, swelling of the nervous tissue, or a critical accumulation of the chemical in the brain. From the clinical viewpoint, this syndrome has been mainly observed in young patients or in patients who exhibit hysterical behavior. In any case, the therapy employed gives us no hint as to the etiology of this state: positive results have been described following psychotherapy, or parenteral treatment with sedatives, stimulants, and antiparkinsonian agents. As a matter of fact, the crises are labile and transitory, and they may disappear even if the doses of the neuroleptic are increased.

The parkinsonian syndrome appears usually after one to two weeks of treatment. Indeed, the syndrome closely resembles the neurology of Parkinson's disease, as muscular hypertonia, tremors, and hyperreflexia are present. The individual response plays an important role in the appearance of these side effects; it seems established that this kind of reaction is most common in women. As already stated, the antipsychotic effect is concomitant with hyperkinetic and hypertonic symptoms; therefore, this syndrome was considered as an indicator of the forthcoming antipsychotic benefit. Criteria were developed, such as the "writing test," which is a sensitive, rapid indicator of rigidity and muscular incoordination, to evaluate the advent of the akinetic phenomena (Haase and Janssen, 1965). Even if the therapeutic outcome does not always correlate with the motor phenomena, this test is useful for the regulation of the dosage of the neuroleptic, leading to the optimal balance between motor deficits and therapeutic benefit (Figure 1.4). A further elaboration of this method has been undertaken by some authors (Figure 1.5), who use the measurement of the handwriting area to monitor not only the action of neuroleptics but also of other treatment modalities, such as L-DOPA on parkinsonian patients (Knopp et al., 1970).

The third side effect of neuroleptic therapy is akathisia accompanied by tasikinesia, which usually appear in patients already showing parkinsonism. This syndrome is overtly expressed in motor activity, such as walking, rubbing hands, cleaning, and other automatisms. This behavior is triggered by an irresistible impulse, which

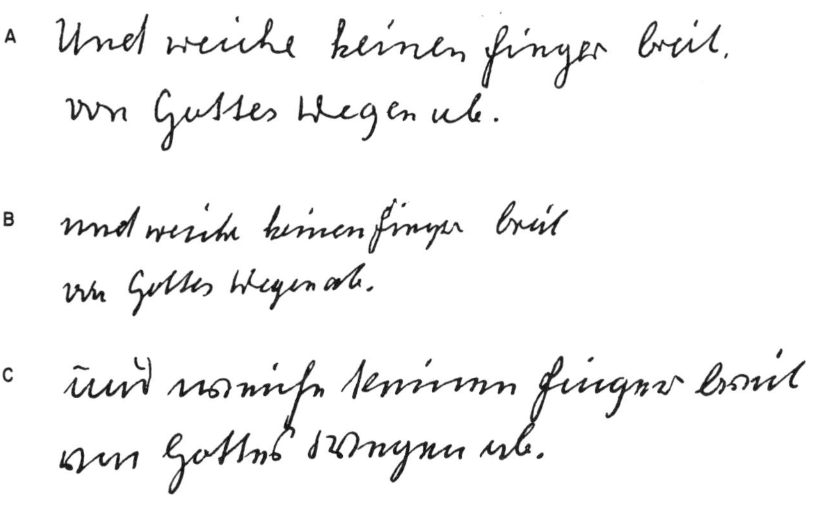

Figure 1.4
Example of the handwriting test used by Haase to monitor the action of neuroleptic drugs. The subject is instructed to copy a simple text (usually a well-known motto or a nursery rhyme). The test is repeated at various intervals in the course of treatment. **(a)** Before treatment. **(b)** During treatment with 10 mg butyrylperazine. **(c)** After discontinuation (from Haase and Janssen, 1965).

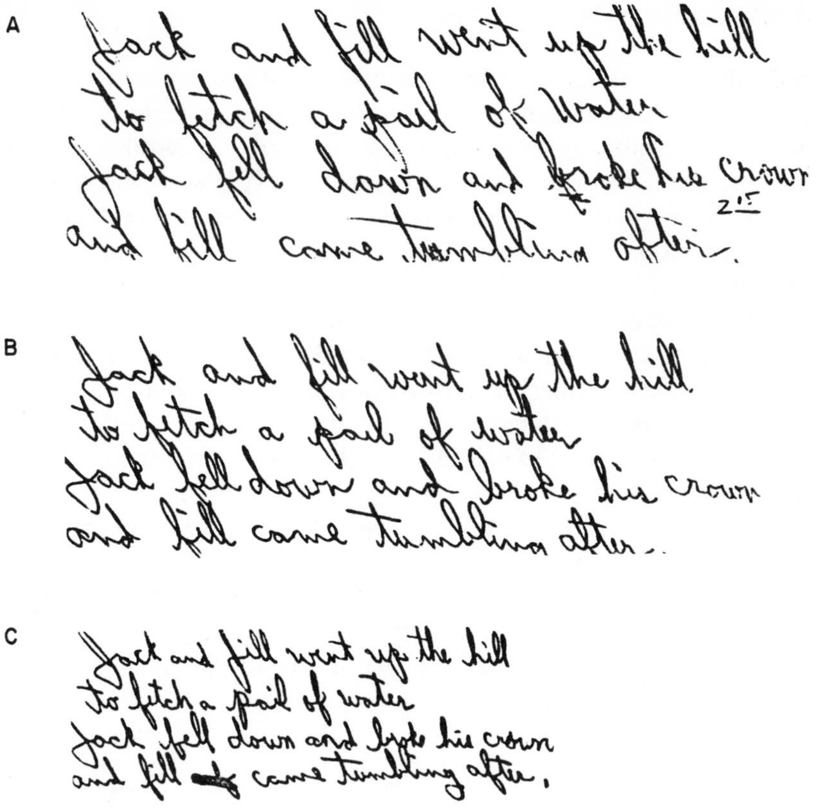

Figure 1.5
The handwriting test was further elaborated by Knopp et al., who measured the handwriting area with a planimeter and displayed the planimetric measurement in graphs as an indicator of clinical response. **(a)** Before treatment. **(b)** Two days later, the patient has received a total of 25 mg of trifluoperazine. **(c)** Four days later, after a total of 85 mg. (From Knopp, 1967.)

depends upon psychic or proprioceptive stimuli; the patient frequently complains about discomfort in his joints or extremities.

Beyond doubt, these three groups of disturbances depend on the extrapyramidal system, as the various manifestations clearly follow the classic descriptions of degenerative or postencephalic parkinsonism. It should be added in this context that, besides its motor component, true Parkinson's disease affects also the psyche and mentation and is characterized by sedation and depression; these symptoms also resemble those due to the phenothiazines. It is obvious that these drugs alter the functioning of the extrapyramidal system, inducing complex phenomena that include both motor and psychic symptoms. Accordingly, a psychological theory of the action of phenothiazines has been suggested that considers the effect of the drugs on the "extrapyramidal psychokinetic conation" (Haase and Janssen, 1965). *Conation* is held to be a psychophysical entity that is the source of each of our acts. Schizophrenia would thus be concomitant to an alteration of the conation, leading to aberrant behavior and aberrant mentation. The neuroleptics, affecting this abnormal conation, block it, and in view of the indivisible character of the conation, they produce simultaneous motor and psychic effects.

Among other side effects described for these drugs, one is particularly worthy of mention because it gave rise to an unusual therapeutic application. Several phenothiazines, and especially thioridazine, inhibit ejaculation but do not impair potency or orgasm. There are favorable reports on the use of this drug in cases of premature ejaculation and nocturnal emission (Mellgren, 1967).

Effects on Animals

When the psychotropic effects of CPZ, which were exciting and novel at the time, were demonstrated in the clinic, CPZ, as well as related substances, were sent back to the laboratory for a reevaluation.

Pharmacologists realized that the methods available to them were not sufficiently refined for the evaluation of the central effects of drugs. In the search for new approaches, they had to invade the fields of neurophysiology and psychology; soon they were recording the electrical activity of the brain and applying such methods of experimental psychology as operant conditioning in their effort to analyze the effects of the psychotropic drugs. Biochemical investigations also gained in prominence: in particular, the influence of psychotropic agents on cerebral chemical transmitters was studied. These developments were so plentiful that it is impossible to present in any detail the laboratory experiments with phenothiazines. We shall attempt instead to stress those effects that, at least to some degree, characterize their action. These will be discussed in relation to behavioral, EEG, and biochemical changes.

Behavioral Effects. At certain doses, all phenothiazines depress spontaneous activity, induce muscular hypotonia, and cause somnolence; at higher doses, a catatonic state appears. This is in agreement with the clinical results, which indicate a lytic effect of CPZ on certain spastic states and, on the other hand, the appearance of extrapyramidal disturbances such as dystonia, parkinsonism, and akathisia. Certain motor effects of CPZ appear immediately upon treatment, and others appear some time after treatment. Among the immediate symptoms, there is lowering of muscle tone. Research aimed at clarifying this phenomenon has dealt with the effect of CPZ on spinal and supraspinal reflexes, on decerebrate rigidity, on facilitation and inhibition of motor activity due to electrical stimulation of some cerebral areas and (most significantly) of the reticular formation. CPZ action seemed generally depressant on both monosynaptic and polysynaptic spinal reflexes. Detailed investigations in animals with lesions at various levels of the cerebrospinal axis proved that this inhibition depended upon the action of the substance on the higher centers, as it could not be obtained in spinal animals. The reticular formation is probably the site of action of CPZ, since experiments dealing with electrical stimulation of facilitatory and inhibitory areas of the brainstem have demonstrated that the drug produces a significant depression of the modulatory influences of these areas on lower motoneurones (Killam, 1968).

Decerebrate rigidity is also influenced by CPZ. Increased muscle tone is obtained in animals (usually cats) either with a midcollicular prepontine transection (the so-called Sherrington preparation) or with ligature of the carotid and vertebral arteries (the so-called Pollock-Davis or anemic decerebration). In the midcollicular preparation, rigidity is due to the hyperactivity of the gamma motoneuronal loop; in the anemic preparation, rigidity is produced by a direct excitation of the alpha motor system. Henatsch and Ingvar (1956) pointed out the differential effect of CPZ on these two types of rigidity; they found that doses of CPZ releasing the midcollicular rigidity did not influence the anemic preparation. According to Randall and Schallek (1968), CPZ is also effective on the anemic preparation, but at much higher doses. These observations may be relevant to the clinical findings that point to the influence of CPZ on spastic disorders.

Another immediate effect of CPZ is sedation; this effect is very clearly illustrated by the blockade of the "sham rage" induced by cortical ablation or by specific cerebral lesions. The violent, purposeless, and inappropriate reaction to slight stimulation observed in diencephalic cats is suppressed by small doses (0.1 mg/kg) of the drug, doses that hardly influence the behavior of intact animals (Dasgupta et al., 1954). The sedative effect of CPZ was studied also on the hyperactive behavior produced by some stimulant drugs (amphetamines, apomorphine, cocaine). The stereotyped activity produced by amphetamine in the rat (sniffing, licking, biting) is strongly antagonized by CPZ and other phenothiazines. This technique has been described as highly specific for the screening of neuroleptic drugs, since other sedatives such as meprobamate, chlordiazepoxide, and the barbiturates are much less specific in this regard (Munkvad et al., 1968).

Other behavioral effects of CPZ were studied through careful observation of general patterns of behavior, like sociability, contentment, excitement, aggressive or defensive hostility, and so forth. It is of interest that CPZ seems to influence behavior connected with high-energy activity, like aggression, more than low-energy activity, like brooding. However, CPZ does not always tame; for instance, docile monkeys and dogs may respond to the drug with an increase in aggressiveness.

One of the most salient delayed effects of the drug is catalepsy (Courvoisier et al., 1957). This syndrome occurs a certain time (from one to four hours) after administration of high doses; it has been described for all the antipsychotic phenothiazines, especially for the piperazine derivatives (Morpurgo and Theobald, 1964). Daily administration of small, subcataleptigenic doses of the drugs gives rise to catalepsy, after a certain number of days (Boissier and Simon, 1964). Many authors therefore consider that this phenomenon could be related to the parkinsonism induced by these drugs in man. This theory is further supported by the finding (Morpurgo, 1962) that the antiparkinsonian drugs (scopolamine, trihexyphenidyl) antagonize this syndrome. Very likely, the phenothiazines, in addition to their immediate effects (which can be explained as due to a competition with the central neurotransmitters, most probably norepinephrine and dopamine) also exhibit a delayed effect on the storage, transport, and turnover of these neurohormones; this effect leads to motor symptoms entirely different from those that appear immediately after treatment. It is this particular effect that bears upon the mechanisms responsible for the antipsychotic activity, as the antipsychotic effects in man are delayed and accompanied by the symptoms of extrapyramidal deficit.

Keeping in mind this two-stage action of CPZ, let us consider some of its other effects, particularly those on conditioning. The experiments in this area are particularly numerous, and a number of phenothiazines were tested on various types of conditioning: avoidance, reward, conditioned emotional responses, and so forth. It appears that the phenothiazines that are therapeutically effective as antipsychotics are particularly effective in blocking avoidance conditioning, as the following example will show. Rats were trained to climb up a vertical pole when they heard a warning sound that preceded a shock; after appropriate dosages of CPZ derivatives, the rats failed to respond to the warning but still responded to the shock (Courvoisier et al., 1957). (See Figures 1.6, 1.7, and 1.8) The drugs have a similar effect on another shock-avoidance response produced by training in a shuttle or jumping box, where rats (or dogs) learn to avoid shock from a grid floor by jumping over a barrier when they hear a warning sound. Fully trained animals lose this learned ability when they are treated with CPZ (Janssen et al., 1966). Under other experimental conditions, such as reward situations or conditioned emotional responses, CPZ and other phenothiazines proved to have less effect. Because a tolerance develops to the drugs among the animals conditioned to avoid shock, a parallel between the antipsychotic effect and the influence on conditioned behavior is questionable.

EEG Effects. Another area that has been the subject of many investigations is that of the effects of phenothiazines on cerebral electrical activity. One of the first EEG studies was that of Longo et al. (1954), carried out in the rabbit. These authors described a characteristic "synchronizing" action of the drug, manifested by the appearance of patterns of slow activity, consisting of 2–3 c/sec waves, 8–12 c/sec spindles, and of 7 c/sec waves with a slow ascending phase. These modifications appear after administration of doses varying from 1–5 mg/kg.

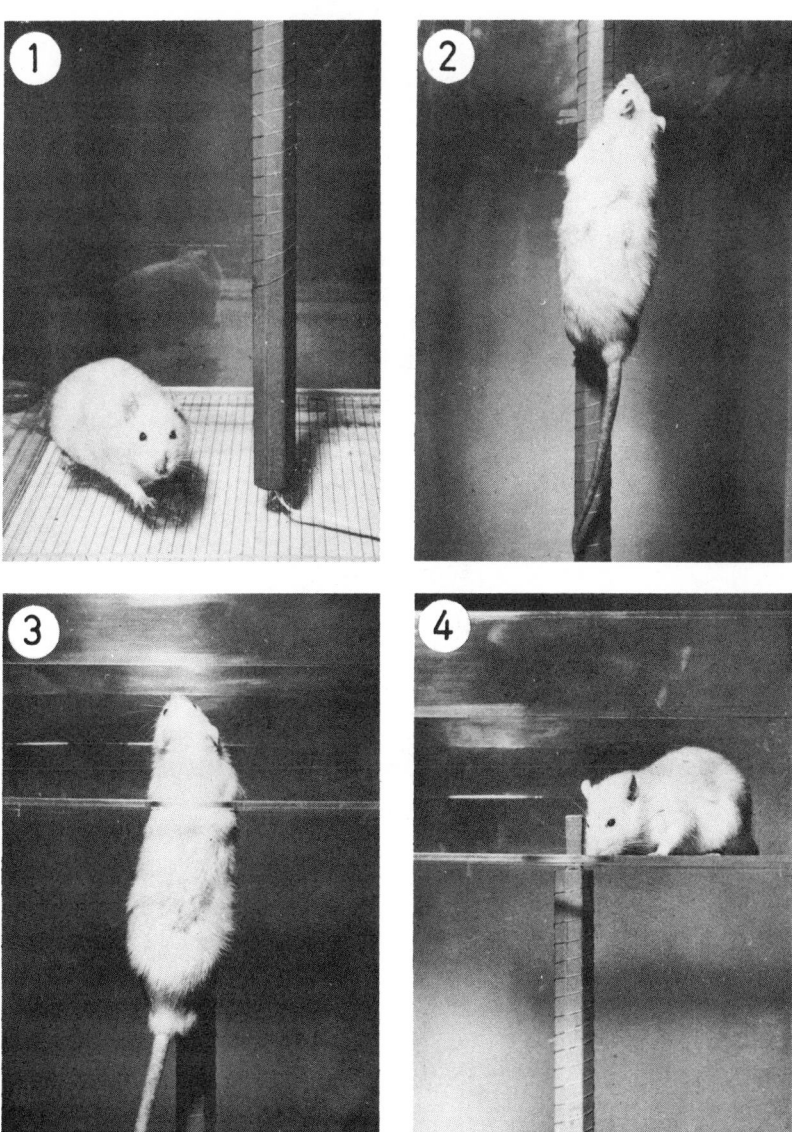

Figure 1.6
The effects of chlorpromazine on avoidance conditioning are demonstrated by the
pole-climbing method. A rat is taught to climb a pole when the floor of the cage is
electrified (unconditioned stimulus); then the animal learns to climb a pole at the
sound of a buzzer (conditioned stimulus). The photographs show the performance of
a conditioned animal. Various refinements of the basic setup have been introduced.
(From Gatti and Frank, 1961.)

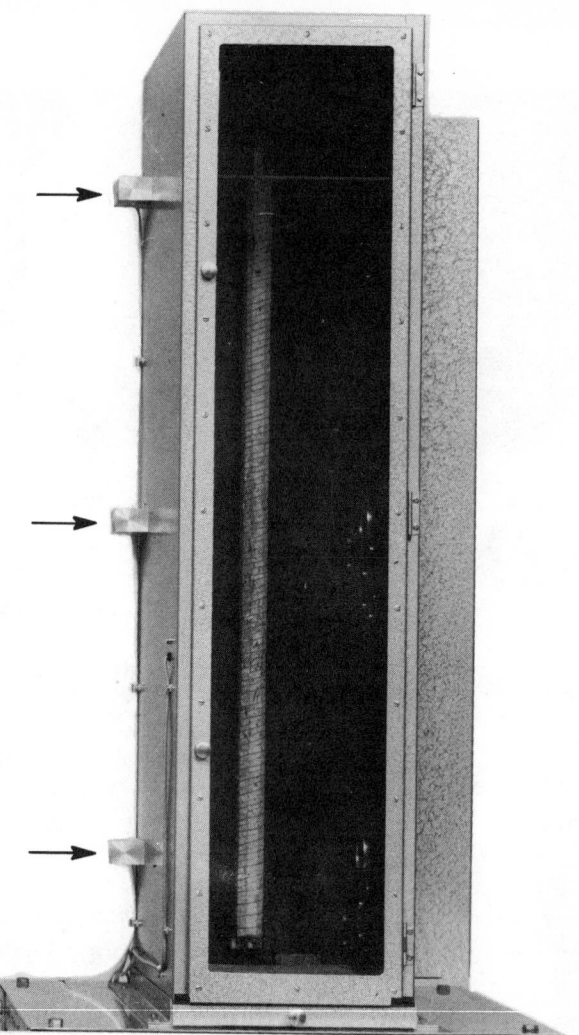

Figure 1.7
In this photograph, three photoelectric cells can be seen
(*arrows*), which give the speed of climbing, registered in a
kimograph (Figure 1.8). (From Gatti and Frank, 1961.)

Longo et al. assigned this "synchronization" of the cortical
rhythms to a depression of the reticular activating system. It should
be remembered that at the time CPZ was studied, this system had
just received a great deal of scrutiny from the neurophysiologists
(Moruzzi and Magoun, 1949). The reticular formation is a medially

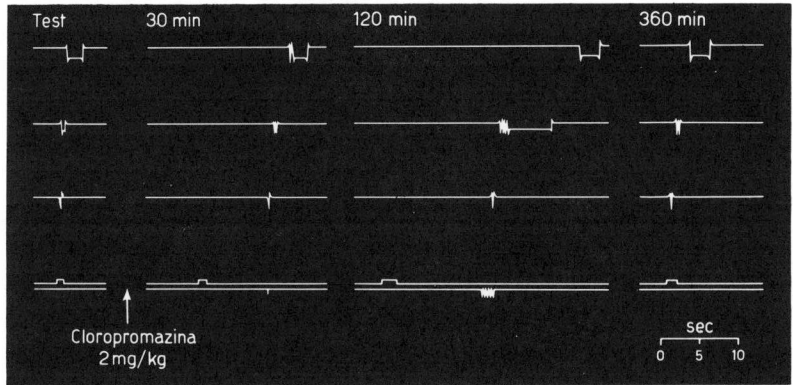

| Test | 30 min | 120 min | 360 min |

Cloropromazina
2mg/kg

sec
0 5 10

Figure 1.8
A record of the behavior of a rat in the setup shown in Figures 1.6 and 1.7, demonstrating the effects of CPZ. In the lower tracing are inscribed the sound of the buzzer (*upper deflection*) and the delivery of the shock (*downward deflection*). Administration of the drug first delays (30 min.) and later blocks (120 min.) the conditioned response. At the time shown, the escape response is still present when the unconditioned stimulus (electrification of the grid floor) is presented, but the climbing is slower. The performance comes back to normal 360 minutes after treatment (from Gatti and Frank, 1961, modified).

located multisynaptic neural network that extends from the lower level of the pons to the ventromedial thalamus. This neural network receives collateral fibers from ascending sensory pathways; unlike sensory input to the pyramidal tract, sensory input to the reticular formation does not retain its distinct identity, as there is no segregation of the incoming fibers. Experiments employing stimulations, lesions, and recording of the electrical activity provided evidence for the concept that the reticular formation controls several manifestations of motor and autonomic activities as well as electrogenesis, and that it elaborates upon stimuli coming both from the periphery and from the rostral portions of the brain (Figure 1.9). For instance, electrical stimulation of the reticular formation induces an EEG activation, both at cortical and subcortical level, which presents striking similarities to the activation observed during the aroused state; on the other hand, destruction of the reticular formation brings about a state of unresponsiveness—even coma. Thus, the reticular formation was considered to be a specific network responsible for maintaining the EEG and behavioral arousal; hence the term "reticular activating system." For many years, the reticular

ROSTRAL INFLUENCES
on Cerebral Hemisphere

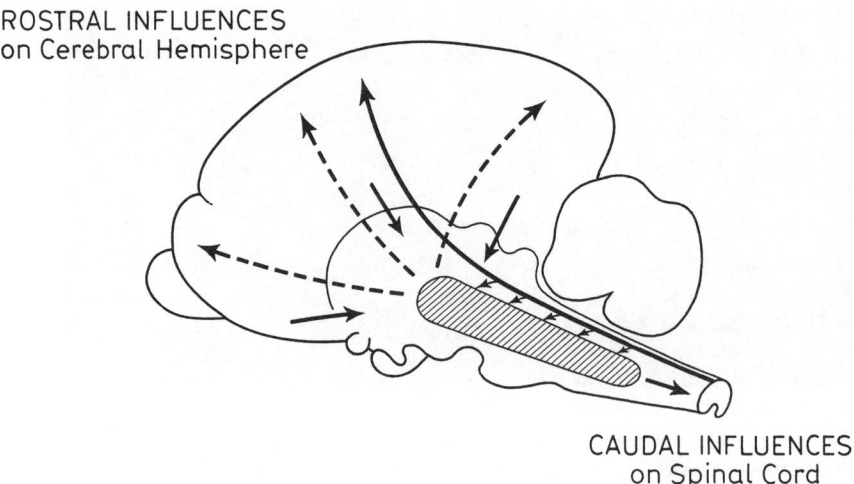

CAUDAL INFLUENCES
on Spinal Cord

Figure 1.9
These functions were attributed to the reticular activating system in the early fifties:
    The reticular system (*striped area*) receives collaterals from the sensory pathways (*continuous arrow*) destined for the postcentral region. The impulses received from the sensory path are integrated and sent to the entire cortex (*broken arrows*), provoking a general *alerting*, or *activation*. In turn, the reticular system can be influenced by impulses originating in the rostral areas (*short arrows*). The caudal influences include facilitating and/or inhibiting effects on spinal reflexes. (See also Figure 3.8.)

formation was considered the target organ of many drugs, in particular, of the neuroleptics. When further investigations were carried out, we witnessed an evolution of our concepts on the functions of this system, which proved to be much more complex than originally thought (see Chapter 3).

Much work was devoted to the EEG effects of the phenothiazines, and to CPZ in particular (for references, see Longo, 1962; Killam, 1962). Although the data were obtained under varied experimental conditions, in different animal species, and on various neurophysiological preparations, they confirmed the "synchronizing" action of the drug, described in the early studies. Yet, upon the administration of high doses (10 mg/kg and up), some authors have observed a desynchronizing effect in the rabbit and in the cat, and have even observed the onset of rhinencephalic seizures. Concomitantly with these EEG modifications, the EEG-activating response evoked by a wide variety of sensory stimuli is generally abolished or depressed, although a few exceptions have been noted. The influence of electrical stimulation of the reticular formation on the activating response has also been studied. Both in the cat and in the rabbit, CPZ reduces the duration of, or blocks completely, the EEG arousal. The effects on the amplitude of single responses evoked in the reticular formation by various kinds of stimuli were inconsistent; the diminution in amplitude described by some authors was not confirmed by other authors. On this particular subject, the reader is referred to a review of Killam (1968).

Compounds closely related to CPZ have also been studied. There is little evidence of differences, except in potency. A comparative study of some phenothiazine derivatives carried out in rabbits bearing chronically implanted electrodes has resulted in the classification of their effects on the cerebral electrical activity, shown in Table 1.1. These compounds have been used in human

Table 1.1 *Action of Some Phenothiazine Derivatives on the EEG and Its Activation*

Drug	Synchronization	Block of the Activation
Levomepromazine	1.0	1.0
Chlorpromazine	2–3	2–3
Promethazine	3.0	4–5
Prochlorperazine	5.0	5.0
Ethopropazine	5.0	5–10
Diethazine	5.0	10.0

NOTE: Data obtained in cross-experiments with chronically implanted rabbits. Doses in mg/kg, i.v. (From Longo, 1962.)

therapy in a wide range of cases, including parkinsonism, behavioral disorders, and agitated psychomotor states. Considering the relationships between their effects on the cerebral electrogenesis and the clinical data, it should be noted that the greater the effect of a given compound on the EEG, the more effective its sedative properties in humans. In other words, the EEG "synchronization" seems related to the sedative action of the drugs but has only limited significance with regard to the long-range influence on psychopathological states.

It should be stressed, however, that in these experiments, as well as in the majority of the studies found in the literature, animals were injected with either one dose or a series of doses, all given in one experimental day; therefore, an extrapolation of the results to long-range effects in man is at least questionable. On the other hand, few investigations have considered the effect of chronic administration of these agents, and the available results are contradictory. In the rabbit, daily administration of several phenothiazines provokes a trend toward EEG activation (Doyle et al. 1968); in cats treated for three weeks with thioridazine and thioproperazine Borenstein et al. (1969) noted an increase in slow-wave sleep. Further research along these lines is highly desirable.

The antiemetic effect of CPZ is an example of close parallelism of human and animal data; all the phenothiazines exhibit a potent antagonistic effect upon apomorphine emesis in the dog. While the emetic centers may be considered anatomically as part of the caudal reticular formation, the antiemetic effect of the phenothiazines does not parallel their synchronizing effect. In fact, according to Longo (1962), prochlorperazine, a potent antiemetic, is less active than several other phenothiazines with regard to its EEG effects.

Biochemical Research

As can be seen from this short presentation, it seems that the phenothiazines produce various and seemingly unrelated actions, suggesting a widespread biochemical influence. It should be remembered that the first studies on CPZ revealed its many autonomic effects. If, on one hand, the antiadrenergic, anticholinergic, antihistaminic, and antiserotoninic properties of this drug caused confusion and rendered its classification difficult, on the other hand, they implied a wide range of biological activities: the original trade name, Largactil, makes obvious reference to these properties.

Subsequent biochemical investigations confirmed this notion as they demonstrated the capacity of this drug to influence almost all enzyme-directed processes; the major part of these studies dealt with *in vitro* experiments and will not be summarized here; the reader is referred to general reviews of the subject, such as that of Guth and Spirtes (1964). Although caution must be exercised with regard to the transference of *in vitro* data to the study of the living body, it is nevertheless true that biochemical investigations on the various phenothiazines have contributed significantly to our knowledge of their action. A fact that emerges from these and related studies is that these drugs affect the permeability of the cellular and subcellular membranes. We do not know to what extent this effect can be dissociated from the effect on enzymes—in fact, the membrane action necessarily involves enzymes, and the reverse is also true. This influence upon membrane can explain the antiedemic and anti-inflammatory action (which was shown to be independent of the antihistaminic properties of the drugs) as well as the inhibition of intestinal absorption of various substances. Similarly, in regard to the central nervous system, studies with labeled compounds demonstrated the effect of various phenothiazines on brain uptake of sodium, potassium, and sulfur.

Research on the turnover and content of central neurotransmitters has demonstrated that several antipsychotic phenothiazines increase the turnover rate of the catecholamines. The increased production of catecholamines is thought to be due to an attempt to overcome the receptor block induced by these substances. Whether this action is important for the antipsychotic effect of these drugs remains to be established (see Andén et al., 1970).

RESERPINE

Primitive East Indian medicine frequently employed the root of an Apocynaceous shrub, *Rauwolfia serpentina*. Therapeutic applications of the extracts and decoctions of this plant were variable and imprecise, as one could expect in folk medicine. Yet, the use of rauwolfia in agitation, madness, and hypertension was frequent. This medium-size plant (1 yard high, with whitish flowers and long twisting roots) grows in India, Ceylon, and Malaysia. It was named after Rauwolf, a 16th-century botanist, who visited Africa and Asia to study medicinal plants.

Around 1930, the therapeutic properties of this plant attracted the attention of Indian investigators, who published numerous articles both on the extraction and identification of the active principles of rauwolfia and on clinical studies, particularly with regard to the therapy of hypertension and of states of anxiety and insomnia. Several alkaloids were extracted from the roots, including ajmaline, serpentine, and serpentinine. Pharmacological studies did not show any evidence of a calming property of any of these three compounds.

In 1950, the first total extracts of the root were introduced in the West in the therapy of hypertension; the results were encouraging. At the same time chemical research was carried out to ascertain the active principles of rauwolfia, and in 1952 CIBA investigators isolated from the oleoresin of the root a series of alkaloids, reserpine being one of them. Like the other alkaloids isolated earlier, reserpine has a relatively complicated yohimbinoid skeleton (Figure 1.10); related alkaloids which were isolated were deserpidine, rescinamine,

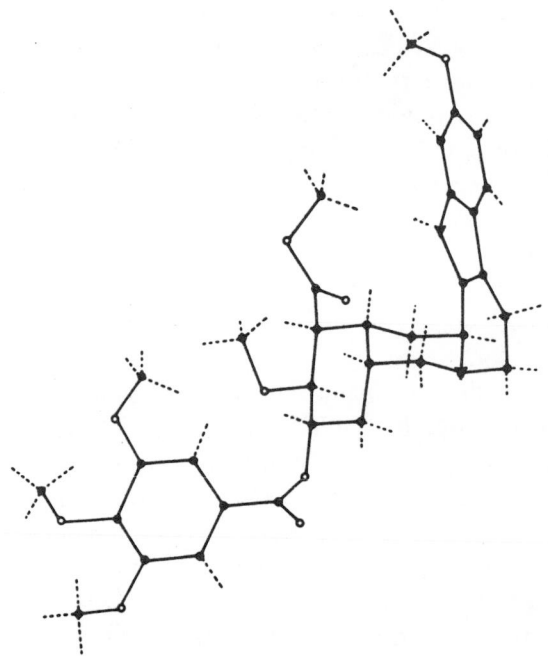

Figure 1.10
Stereochemical diagram of a reserpine molecule. Intensive investigations have led to the identification of the conformational structure of reserpine. The spatial arrangement of atoms and groups in the molecule is critical for its biological effect. Dots represent carbon atoms, circles oxygen atoms, and triangles nitrogen atoms. (From Schlitter and Plummer, 1964. Courtesy of Academic Press.)

raunescine, and pseudoreserpine. The immediate therapeutic application of reserpine was, like that of the total extract, in arterial hypertension; the first symposium dedicated to reserpine emphasized this particular use of reserpine (Miner, 1954). All the researchers who at that time conducted comparative studies on both the extract and reserpine itself agreed that reserpine was responsible for the major part of the therapeutic effectiveness of the extract, that this action appeared only after a delay, and that the lowering of blood pressure was accompanied by sedation. This latter observation, as well as the reports in the Indian literature, directed attention towards the possibility of applying this drug in the therapy of neuropsychiatric states. In fact, the symposium mentioned above contained the first report on clinical effects, in controlled experiments, of both the extract and the alkaloid, which were given to schizophrenics and other psychotic patients (Kline, 1954). The prudent conclusion of Kline was that reserpine was an effective sedative that could be used in psychiatric clinics for the treatment of anxiety and obsessive compulsive drives.

Effects on Man

The results of the first studies of antipsychotic effects of reserpine were rather controversial (Miner, 1955). It should be remembered in this context that chlorpromazine was introduced in the clinic at the same time, and investigators used the same approach and looked for the same results from each drug; in fact, they were after analogies that did not exist. In these first studies, massive doses of reserpine (up to 60 mg daily) were given to patients in an attempt to find a clear-cut, immediate effect. Only after additional progress in these studies did it become clear that clinical improvement occurred with much lower dosages and after a delay varying from one to three weeks.

Today the dose range of reserpine for the treatment of psychotic conditions varies between 5 and 10 mg daily, and is usually given orally. In the first days of treatment, while patients tend to become more relaxed, drowsy, and inactive, there is no obvious change in their pathological thoughts or feelings. Some patients react during treatment with restlessness, insomnia, and exacerbation of the anxiety-tension state, and this response unfavorably impressed the clinicians during the early trials. If, however, treatment is continued, a gradual improvement is noticed, with a reversal of the psychotic disturbances, increased sociability, and amenability to psychotherapy—results very similar to those observed with the phenothiazines.

This antipsychotic effect is accompanied by many side actions. The autonomic disturbances depend upon the increased parasympathetic and decreased sympathetic activity, and include hypotension, bradycardia, flushing, and nasal congestion; activation of peptic ulcers or acute gastric erosion have also been reported. Neurological and psychic effects include parkinsonism (without the dystonic crisis) and depression, which is the most serious reaction. The drug also engenders an unpleasant mood when given in small doses in the course of nonpsychiatric treatment and is counterindicated in susceptible individuals, in whom it may exaggerate suicidal tendencies. Other side effects involve the endocrine system: loss of libido, impotence, and gynecomastia in men, lactation in women. Reserpine is also an antagonist of thyroxin and has been used therapeutically in hyperthyroidism.

The wide range of side effects, the preliminary exacerbation of delusions and hallucinations, and the lesser activity in comparison with the phenothiazine derivatives contributed to progressive curtailment of the clinical use of reserpine (Shepherd et al., 1968). However, it is still employed when patients are resistant to other forms of treatment.

Effects on Animals

The same uncertainties described for the clinical trials were encountered by those engaged in animal research. The researchers knew that they were dealing with an extremely effective substance that exhibited a variety of actions, both central and peripheral—actions that were difficult to classify. The acute toxicity of reserpine was relatively low, and the lethal effect appeared only after a delay. The mechanism of toxicity itself was not readily explainable. In the dog, for instance, death was attributed to dehydration, caused by the intense and prolonged diarrhea.

In view of reserpine's clinical efficacy in hypertensive states, its influence on the cardiovascular system was studied extensively. No peripheral sympatholytic or parasympatholytic activity was exhibited by the drug, and there was no evidence of ganglionic blockade. Only a modest drop in blood pressure was observed in the unanesthetized animals; a more marked fall was obtained, after a certain delay, in animals under barbiturate anesthesia. On the other hand, the most obvious effect of reserpine was the production of a state of quietitude and sedation, and the photographs of the treated monkey in the original papers of CIBA investigators remain a classical documentation of this taming effect (Plummer et al., 1954). The effect occurs after a period of about one hour; although the animal loses its vicious behavior and remains quiet, it is readily aroused and eats normally (Figure 1.11). The sedative action of the alkaloid was confirmed in other laboratory animals; additional effects observed were miosis, relaxation of the nictitating membrane, and augmentation of the secretory and motor activity of the gastrointestinal tract. All these results suggested that a central site of action was very likely, and the symptoms were attributed to a "paralysis" of the central sympathetic system with a resulting increase in parasympathetic activity.

We owe the initiation of more cogent investigations of the mechanism of action of reserpine to Brodie and his collaborators (Pletscher et al., 1955). These authors observed both *in vivo* and *in vitro* a reduction in tissue content of serotonin following treatment with reserpine. This depletion was also observed in the brain; in the *in vivo* experiments, the serotonin metabolite 5-hydroxyindolacetic acid appeared in the urine. On the basis of these results, Brodie suggested that serotonin reduction was intimately involved in the various pharmacological effects of reserpine. Subsequently, it was found that reserpine also depletes catecholamines (norepinephrine, dopamine) (Carlsson et al., 1957; Holzbauer and Vogt, 1956). These observations stimulated an immense expansion of research in this field, which further defined the significance, metabolism, and role of these monoamines. For example, the concept of a dynamic equilibrium of the biochemical processes of the organism, advanced many years earlier by Schoenheimer (1942), was reappraised and gained ascendance because this hypothesis could be used to explain many of the biochemical phenomena observed with reserpine and its analogs.

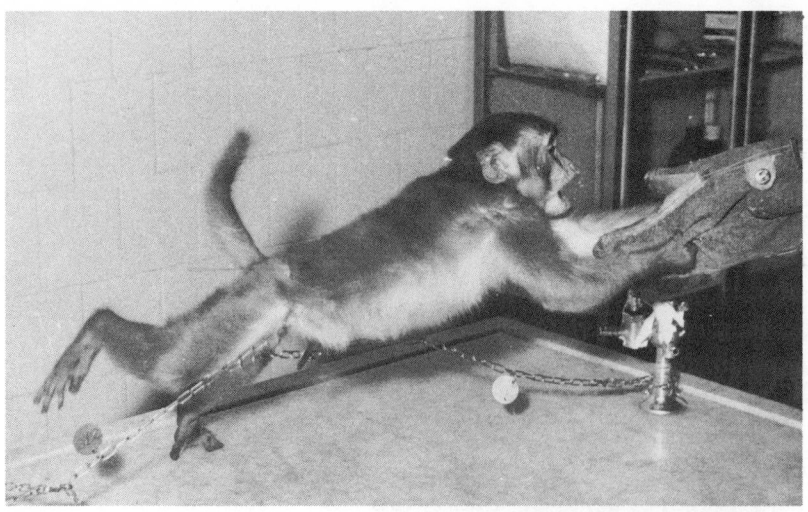

Figure 1.11
Reserpine (1 mg/kg) induces a
state of sedation and tameness in
a Rhesus monkey, which before
treatment (*upper photograph*) was
aggressive and untractable.

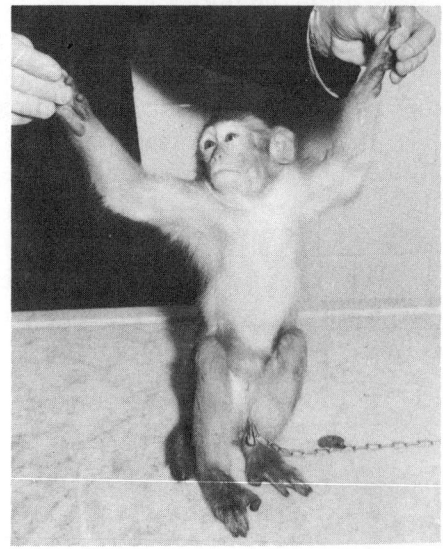

In fact, today monoamines and other substances allegedly involved as transmitters or modulators are not regarded as immobile material, kept in storage until the moment of use; rather, they are believed to be continuously formed, stored, released, and destroyed at the cellular and subcellular levels.

In addition to reserpine and some related natural and semisynthetic analogs, other drugs that diminish the body content of indolamines and catecholamines have been described and studied (Sulser and Bass, 1968). These are: the synthetic benzoquinolines, such as tetrabenazine; the ring-substituted aralkylamines, such as bis-(3-4-dichlorophenethyl)-amine, and prenylamine (Segotin). Other substances, on the other hand, preferentially lower the catecholamine content; these are α-methyl DOPA, and α-methyl-*p*-tyrosine. Still other drugs diminish specifically the serotonin content, such as *p*-chlorophenylalanine and *p*-chlorometamphetamine. The mechanisms of action of these substances was progressively clarified, and it was demonstrated that the depletion of the amines takes place via various mechanisms. Reserpine and tetrabenazine block the intraneuronal storage of the various amines, which are therefore exposed to, and destroyed by, monoamine oxidase (MAO). α-Methyl-*p*-tyrosine inhibits tyrosine hydroxylase and causes a selective reduction of brain catecholamines, leaving serotonin essentially unaffected. α-Methyl DOPA inhibits DOPA decarboxylase and causes a fall of brain dopamine, norepinephrine, *and serotonin*. Serotonin and dopamine return to control level within 24 hours; norepinephrine remains low for several days (Hess et al., 1961). *p*-Chlorophenylalamine (PCPA), a potent inhibitor of tryptophan hydroxylase, blocks the synthesis of serotonin. Of all these substances, only reserpine, and to a lesser extent tetrabenazine, have a proven antipsychotic action. Therefore, if the depletion of the monoamines is linked with this action, the special clinical effectiveness of reserpine and tetrabenazine should be explained by their specific depletion mechanism, the rapid destruction of the amines liberated by these drugs playing a role of particular importance.

With regard to the other substances mentioned, particularly those that selectively decrease either the catecholamines or serotonin, these drugs act as inhibitors of the synthesis; therefore, the lowering of the amine content that they induce is not strictly comparable to that of reserpine.

Reserpine itself still presents certain problems, as it remains unclear whether its tranquilizing action is associated with changes of brain serotonin, brain catecholamines, or is independent from amine depletion. In fact, some reports indicate that correlation between levels of monoamines and behavioral changes in animals is poor. A good example is offered by studies of benzoquinoline derivatives. Tetrabenazine, like reserpine, decreases catecholamines and serotonin content; even though it is less potent and shorter acting, its autonomic and behavioral effects are similar to those of reserpine and are antagonized by MAO inhibitors. Nevertheless, sedation and other depressive effects can also be produced by some other benzo-quinoline derivatives, such as benzoquinamide, which do not change the cerebral amine content; nor is benzoquinamide's behavioral effect antagonized by the MAO inhibitors (Pletscher et al., 1968). In clinical use, benzoquinamide has no antipsychotic effect but rather a sedative action similar to that of the barbiturates (Shepherd et al., 1968).

Other inconsistencies exist in the studies of the action of reserpine on the cerebral electrical activity. Some authors have described a prolonged EEG desynchronization which contrasts with the animal's depression. Other authors have described a biphasic action in the rabbit, consisting of an initial period (30–60 minutes) of desynchronization, followed by a period of synchronization. Still others reported an alternating pattern of desynchronization and synchronization unrelated to the animal's behavior (for references, see Longo 1962). Some observations, made on the cat, pointed to an effect of reserpine that has been interpreted as "rhinencephalic" (Killam and Killam, 1956; Sigg and Schneider, 1957; Passouant et al., 1956). A rapid (20 c/sec), high-voltage activity, having all the characteristics of a convulsive electrical seizure, has been recorded at the level of the dorsal hippocampus and amygdala; this was particularly noticeable following repeated daily administrations of reserpine to animals bearing permanent electrodes. Electrical stimulation of the same area resulted in the lengthening and in the intensification of the convulsive episodes. There were no reports of rhinencephalic seizures in the rabbit (Longo and Napolitano, 1955; Gangloff and Monnier, 1957).

In a reappraisal of the EEG data on the alkaloid, Pscheidt et al. (1964) emphasize that the divergent results may be due to differences in methodology. They have demonstrated that (*a*) when rabbits are treated with reserpine *before* the light ether anesthesia necessary for the implantation of the electrodes, the late period of synchronization is present, and that (*b*) it is not present when animals are injected with the drug *after* the surgery—the latter animals exhibit only continuous activation. The surgical manipulation does not interfere, however, with the depletion of the amines from the brain, which is similar in the two groups of animals. These data cast doubt on the notion that reserpine EEG effects are due to amine depletion: if the first phase of activation depends upon the liberation of some free amines, which are then rapidly destroyed, it is not readily apparent why there should be so much variability in the second phase, which corresponds to the depletion stage.

It is appropriate here to quote other data indicating that a change in the life cycle of the brain amines influences the EEG. PCPA, which affects serotonin specifically, induces in animals an increase of the periods of desynchronization (Jouvet, 1968; Koella et al., 1968); these authors suggested that serotonin may play an important role in the regulation of the sleep-vigilance cycles. Experiments carried out by Karczmar et al. (1970) demonstrated that in reserpinized animals the administration of eserine induces an EEG and behavioral syndrome similar to that of paradoxical sleep (PS). All the phenomenology of this phase of sleep—including cortical activation, hippocampal theta waves, occipital spikes, ocular movements, and relaxation of the neck muscles—could be simulated by combining these two drugs. This "pharmacological model" of PS was obtained in rabbits and cats treated with reserpine (1 mg/kg) and receiving 4–48 hours later eserine (0.1–0.2 mg/kg); since eserine inhibits the brain acetylcholinesterase, thus causing accumulation of acetylcholine, and the effectiveness of eserine in inducing the PS seemed to run parallel to the kinetics of the depleting action of reserpine, Karczmar et al. (1970) hypothesize that accumulation of acetylcholine in the presence of low levels of brain amines may constitute the physiological condition underlying PS.

BUTYROPHENONES

The butyrophenones are compounds endowed with antipsychotic and sedative properties. These drugs, developed in the Janssen laboratories in Belgium, may be considered chemically as derivatives of meperidine, a narcotic analgesic agent (Janssen, 1965a). Some of the butyrophenones constitute an interesting link between the analgesics and the neuroleptics as they exhibit morphine and chlorpromazine-like effects (Figure 1.12).

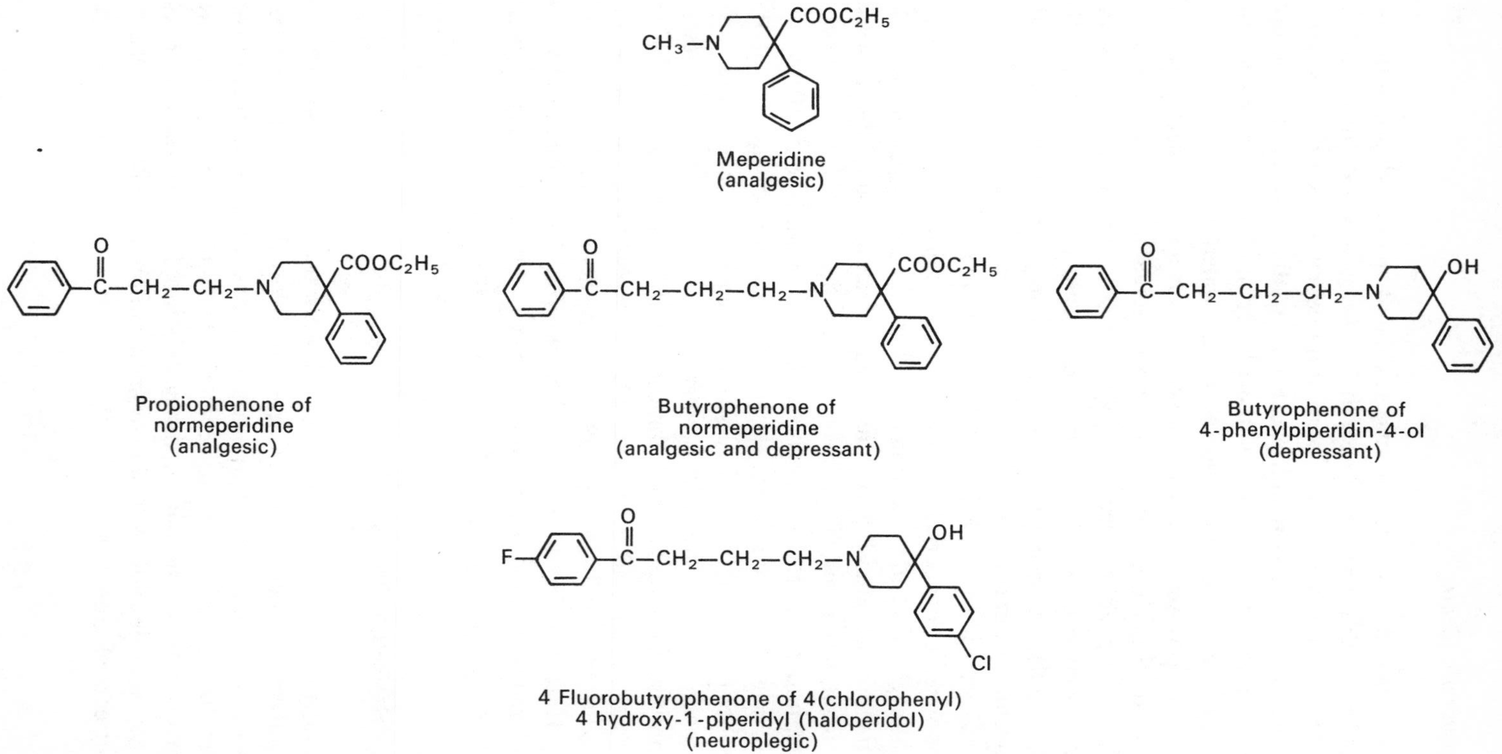

Figure 1.12
Transition from analgesic to neuroleptic activity in a series of derivatives of 4-phenyl-piperidine leading to haloperidol.

The first derivative of the series, haloperidol, was tested in the neuropsychiatric clinic of Liège, and it was found beneficial in psychomotor agitation and in schizophrenic syndromes (Divry et al., 1958). The butyrophenone series was quite prolific: more than twenty compounds were evaluated clinically and at least seven are commercially available. It should be stressed that the most potent neuroleptics known belong to this series. In the clinic, haloperidol is, in may respects, similar to the piperazine phenothiazines as an antipsychotic agent. According to clinical reports (Haase and Janssen, 1965), the drug is most effective on the over-activity, agitation, and paranoid ideation of schizophrenic patients. In view of its potent depressive effect on the motor system, haloperidol is indicated preferentially in psychomotor agitation of various etiologies: manic reactions, alcoholic delirium, and aggressive behavior. Also, haloperidol treatment gives excellent results in Huntington's chorea, hemiballismus, and tics; in particular, it is the drug of choice in rare and difficult-to-manage syndromes like Gilles de la Tourette's disease (Challas and Brauer, 1963) and latah, both characterized by severe motor and verbal tics (grimacing, jerks, incoordination, accompanied by echolalia and coprolalia). Another commercially used butyrophenone is trifluperidol, which has a CF_3 group in the meta position instead of a Cl in the para position. This drug seems to be useful in the treatment of withdrawn and autistic patients. Other derivatives employed in the clinic are methylperidol (moperone), benperidol, fluanisone and droperidol. All these drugs are very potent neuroleptics; the doses employed are very low, as they range from 2–12 mg daily, usually given orally.

The butyrophenones give rise to prominent extrapyramidal side effects and the incidence of these phenomena is quite high. This undesirable feature is one of the reasons that the butyrophenones are not favorably received by some neuropsychiatrists, who hesitate to use drugs that have no real advantage over the available phenothiazines. It should be taken into account, however, that the butyrophenones are devoid, apart from the extrapyramidal effects, of other side effects. For instance, the incidence of chronic toxic reaction, such as skin, eye, and liver reactions associated with long-term therapy is low; autonomic disturbances, such as orthostatic hypotension, are rare; somnolence is less frequent than in the case of other treatments.

Butyrophenones and "Neuroleptanalgesia"

Another clinical application of the butyrophenones is their combined use with analgesics to produce the condition called "neuroleptanalgesia" (NLA).

NLA is a type of anesthesia produced by various combinations of drugs used by anesthetists in preparing patients for major surgery. The "lytic cocktails" proposed by Laborit in the early fifties are typical examples of these combinations; these procedures were modified slowly so as to develop an heroic mixture that combines (*a*) a neuroleptic, to induce depression, apathy, and akinesia, as well as an antiemetic effect, and (*b*) an analgesic, to obtund pain. This combination alone induces some of the modalities of surgical anesthesia, such as analgesia and depression of reflexes, thus protecting against surgical trauma. In the many drug mixtures of this type tested by clinicians, such butyrophenones as fluanisone or droperidol were frequently included because of their high neuroleptic potency and their short onset and short duration of effect. Among the analgesic components of the mixtures, dextromoramide and fentanyl (an acylated 4-anilinopiperidine) proved to be particularly useful (Holderness et al., 1963).

A combination of droperidol and fentanyl is often used to induce NLA. The ratio between the neuroplegic and the analgesic is 50:1, 1 ml of the mixture usually contains 1 mg of droperidol and 0.02 mg of fentanyl. Ten milliliters are administered by slow intravenous injection and, within five to ten minutes, induce sleepiness, a feeling of detachment, and analgesia. Because of the respiratory depression and even apnea that may occur, respiration and the cardiovascular status of the patient should be monitored. Under NLA the patient is more-or-less vigilant, in the sense that he understands directions and questions, which is particularly useful in neurosurgery (pneumoencephalography, stereotaxy).

In other surgical procedures, NLA is usually associated with nitrous oxide (Martin et al., 1967). It should be stressed, however, that some anesthesiologists indulge in some rather strange combinations, adding to the basic mixture diazepam, hydroxydione, hemineurine, and curaromimetic substances (Huguenard, 1968). These procedures have caused perplexity and have been subjected to criticism.

In conclusion, NLA is a particular state that should be distinguished from general anesthesia and that should also be distinguished from the analgesia or the sedation caused by the individual drugs alone; moreover, the condition of the patient under the influence of this treatment has not yet been fully evaluated. However, with careful planning and application, NLA deserves a place among the techniques available to the anesthesiologists today.

Effects on Animals

Since butyrophenones were introduced following phenothiazines, most of the available studies of butyrophenones deal with comparisons of the two series of drugs. It has been shown that butyrophenones and phenothiazines (mainly the potent piperazine derivatives) have many pharmacological properties in common. The butyrophenones antagonize the stereotyped hyperactivity produced by amphetamine, and the "gnawing" produced by apomorphine in the rat. In the dog, antiemetic action is observed with minimal doses. Spiroperidol, effective at a dose of 0.0006 μM/kg, intravenous, is 3000 times more active than chlorpromazine. The various butyrophenones given orally exert a pronounced inhibitory effect on the conditioned shock-avoidance response in the jumping-box test (Janssen et al., 1965b, 1966, 1967). The experiments carried out by these authors used both rats and dogs. Since these drugs are usually administered orally in man, oral versus parenteral effectiveness has been studied. In the dog, the butyrophenone group is more active orally than the corresponding potent phenothiazine derivatives.

These comparative studies have also shown some differences between the two series. It is interesting that moderate but significant signs of central excitation are observed upon administration of small doses of some butyrophenones. This effect, very clear with triperidol and still noticeable with haloperidol, is absent with chlorpromazine. Figure 1.13 illustrates the effect of these three drugs on the exploratory activity of the rat. Increasing the dosage, depressive effects appear, up to catalepsy. At subtoxic doses these drugs, unlike the phenothiazines, provoke convulsions. This excitatory and convulsant component is also seen in man; for instance, insomnia and reactivation of epileptic crisis have been observed in some patients.

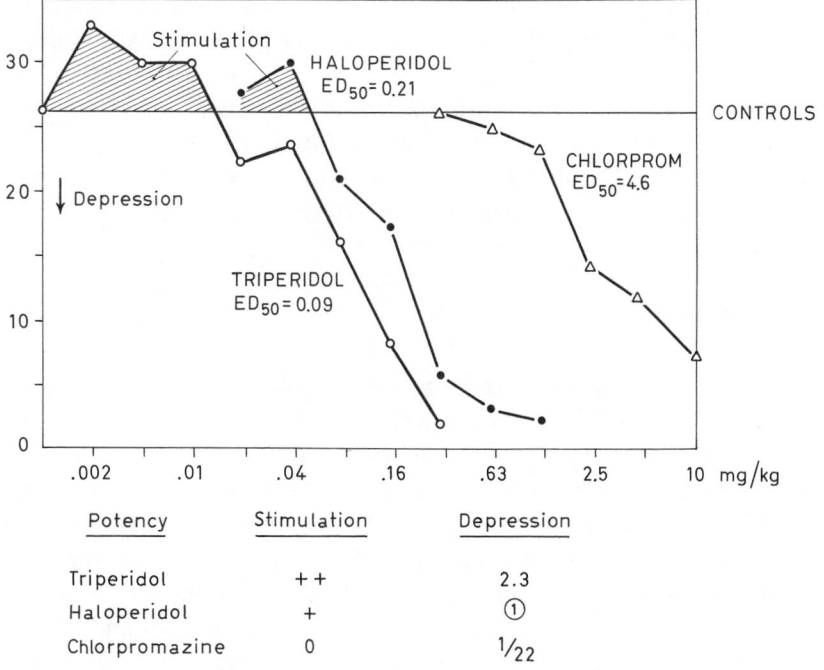

Figure 1.13
Stimulant and depressant effects of two butyrophenones, compared with chlorpromazine, on the exploratory ambulation of rats in an unfamiliar "open-field"
environment. Triperidol is a stronger stimulant than haloperidol; chlorpromazine is a
pure depressant. The rats were submitted to the test four hours after treatment with
the drugs. Ordinates: arbitrary scale of spontaneous activity; abscissae: doses in
mg/kg, s.c. (From Janssen, Symposium Internationale sull'Haloperidol e Triperidol,
Istituto Luso Farmaco, Milano, 1962.)

A great deal of this research has centered on the effects of the
butyrophenones and phenothiazines on the adrenergic and dopaminergic central systems, and some authors have elaborated theories to
explain similarities and differences between these two groups of
drugs, postulating different affinities for the two systems. Janssen
(1967) has proposed a theory on the central action of the butyrophenones. His premise is that these compounds, as well as the phenothiazines (see page 126), tend to decrease the permeability of a
variety of biological membranes and that they exert this effect in
minute concentration. In the central system, the permeability of
membranes for the catecholamines is decreased by the neuroleptic
molecules: the dopaminergic system is the most sensitive to the

drugs. The potent antiemetic effect of butyrophenones, the block of stereotyped behavior (gnawing) and the inhibition of learned avoidance responses are explained through an effect of the drugs on the emetic trigger zone and on the nigrostriatal system, which are largely dopaminergic. The decrease of spontaneous activity and of exploratory movements, the block of operant responding, the cataleptic postures observed with higher doses of butyrophenones are due to an interference with the adrenergic system. Much higher doses are needed to influence other adrenergic areas, such as the vasomotor and the thermoregulating centers. Pronounced peripheral adrenolytic effects likewise do not occur unless the same high doses of the drugs are administered.

Electroencephalographically, the butyrophenones share many common features with the phenothiazines (for references, see Longo and Florio, 1970). Haloperidol, in doses of 0.1–0.2 mg/kg produces in the rabbit synchronization of the EEG and raises the threshold of EEG arousal due to reticular stimulation. Confirming the behavioral data, EEG-seizure activity was observed at doses above 8 mg/kg. In the cat, the synchronizing effect of haloperidol is less evident, yet seizures appear upon administration of high doses. Other derivatives such as triperidol and spiroperidol are more active in modifying the EEG; the latter substance, injected in rabbits in doses of 5–10 μg/kg, modifies the tracing towards synchronization.

Florio and Longo (1971) studied the effects of haloperidol and spiroperidol on the EEG arousal and on the spasm of the head and neck muscles elicited in the rabbit by electrical stimulation of the central gray matter at the mesencephalic level (Figure 1.14). The area stimulated belongs to a pathway (extending from the pons to the thalamus) that is responsible for the so-called tegmental reaction (Ingram et al., 1932); this reaction is a motor response possessing extrapyramidal characteristics and consisting of a turning of the head toward the side being stimulated. Stimulation of this zone probably activates the dopaminergic nigrostriatal system, which plays an important role in the regulation of the postural reflexes. Since the two drugs proved very effective in blocking both the EEG and the motor response to stimulation, these authors attempted to restore the responses by means of various substances (amphetamine, apomorphine, L-DOPA). The intravenous administration of 10–15 mg/kg of L-DOPA produced the reappearance of the EEG desynchronization and the restoration of the spasm of the neck muscles upon stim-

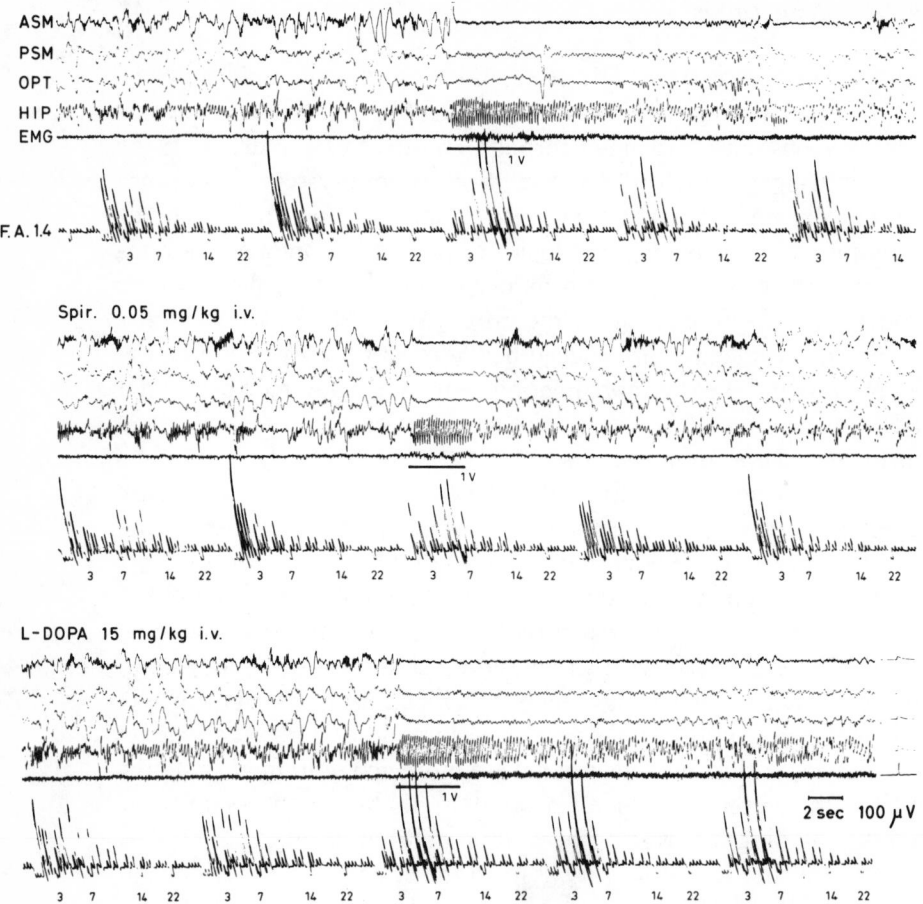

Figure 1.14
Antagonism of L-DOPA on the EEG and motor effects caused by spiroperidol. Acute rabbit preparation.

Upper tracing: control, the stimulation of the mesencephalic periacqueductal gray matter elicits a long-lasting desynchronization of the cortical EEG, appearance of the theta rhythm in the dorsal hippocampus, and spasm of the neck muscles with omo-lateral head rotation (note the increase in voltage of the EMG record).

Spir. 0.05 mg/kg, i.v.: 10 minutes after 0.05 mg/kg of spiroperidol, stimulation of the periacqueductal gray elicits only a short-lasting EEG arousal.

L-DOPA 15 mg/kg, i.v.: 25 minutes after spiroperidol and 10 minutes after L-DOPA 15 mg/kg, i.v., the EEG and motor responses to the stimulation of the periacqueductal gray are fully restored.

Leads: **ASM,** anterior sensorimotor cortex; **PSM,** posterior sensorimotor cortex; **OPT,** optic cortex; **HIP,** dorsal hippocampus; **EMG,** electromyogram of the neck muscles; **FA I-4,** frequency-analysis record of the leads ASM and HIP. (From Florio and Longo, 1971).

ulation (Figure 1.14). Amphetamine and apomorphine, given in intravenous doses of 2–8 mg/kg, caused desynchronization of the EEG, accompanied by signs of behavioral excitation; however, the block of the tegmental response was not antagonized. These results lend weight to the hypothesis that these drugs interfere with the dopaminergic system at the level of the systems responsible for cerebral electrogenesis and for motor responses.

Van Rossum (1967) also attributes the central effects of neuroleptics to a block of the dopaminergic receptors and, in addition, demonstrated an interference between the butyrophenones and dopamine at the periphery. In the dog and the cat, when the sympathomimetic α-receptors are blocked, dopamine causes a lowering of the blood pressure, which is antagonized by some butyrophenones. Van Rossum also considers the problem of the etiology of schizophrenia in this context. If the blockade of the dopaminergic system is in some way correlated with the antipsychotic effect of the drugs of this group, one can postulate that an increased production of dopamine, accompanied by an alteration of its metabolism (thereby causing the formation of abnormal products), could be one of the causative factors of the psychotic syndrome (Stein and Wise, 1971).

This hypothesis can be related to the psychophysical integration theory already discussed (see page 17), and according to which motor regulation and exquisitely psychic processes are tightly connected. The extrapyramidal system, which has been extensively investigated, can be considered the most typical example of this integration, but it should be kept in mind that other discrete systems probably will be included in the future. Some data that support the concept of this integration are the following:

1. Amphethamine, in small doses, causes in the animal and in man psychic and motor excitation and, in larger doses, stereotypes and mental confusion, probably through a direct or indirect stimulation of the catecholaminergic system. If administration of amphetamine is continued for long periods, one notes the occurrence of an "amphetamine psychosis," which is highly similar to the schizophrenic syndrome.

2. The methoxy and methylic derivatives of amphetamine possess psychotomimetic properties (see Chapter 4, Hallucinogenic

Drugs) and moreover can induce catatonia. The cataleptigenic effect is very evident in the methoxyphenylethylamine derivatives, which cause a rigid-hypokinetic syndrome very similar to that observed after bulbocapnine, which has certain structural similarities with these derivatives.

3. Clinical observations indicate that schizophrenia is rarely seen in parkinsonian patients and that schizophrenics who develop parkinsonism usually show marked improvement in their psychotic syndrome (Haase and Janssen, 1965).

References

Andén, N. E., et al. In *The Neuroleptics*, ed. by D. P. Bobon, et al., Karger, Basel, 1970, P. 1.

Boissier, J. R., and Simon, P. *L'Encéphale* 53:109, 1964.

Borenstein, P., et al. *Sem. Hôp. Paris* 45:1271, 1969.

Carlsson, A., et al. *Nature* 180:1200, 1957.

Challas, G., and Brauer, W. *Amer. J. Psychiat.* 120:283, 1963.

Courvoisier, S., et al. *Arch. int. Pharmacodyn.* 92:305, 1953.

Courvoisier, S., et al. In *Psychotropic Drugs*, ed. by S. Garattini and V. Ghetti. Elsevier, Amsterdam, 1957. P. 373.

Dasgupta, S. R., et al. *Arch. int. Pharmacodyn.* 97:149, 1954.

Délay, J., and Deniker, P. *Méthodes Chimiothérapeutiques en Psychiatrie.* Masson, Paris, 1961.

Divry, P., et al. *Acta Neurol. Belg.* 58:878, 1958.

Domino, E. F., et al. In *Drugs Affecting the Central Nervous System*, Vol. 2, ed. by A. Burger. Dekker, New York, 1968. P. 327.

Doyle, C., et al. *Int. J. Neuropharmacol.* 7:87, 1968.

Efron, D. H., ed. *Psychopharmacology. A Review of Progress.* U.S. Dept. of Health, Education and Welfare, Washington, D.C., 1968. P. 2.

Florio, V., and Longo, V. G. *Neuropharmacology* 10:45, 1971.

Freyhan, F. A. *Amer. J. Psychiat.* 115:577, 1959.

Gangloff, H., and Monnier, M. *Helv. Physiol. Acta* 15:83, 1957.

Gatti, G. L., and Frank, M. In *Neuropsychopharmacology*, Vol. II, ed. by E. Rothlin. Elsevier, Amsterdam, 1961. Pp. 147–149.

Guth, P. S., and Spirtes, M. A. *Int. Rev. Neurobiol.* 7:231, 1964.

Haase, H. J., and Janssen, P. A. J. *The Action of Neuroleptic Drugs.* North-Holland, Amsterdam, 1965.

Henatsch, H. D., and Ingvar, D. H. *Arch. Psychiat. Nerv. Krankh.* 195:77, 1956.

Hess, S. M., et al. *J. Pharmacol.* 134:129, 1961.

Holderness, M. C., et al. *Anesthesiology* 24:336, 1963.

Hollister, L. E. *Ann. Rev. Pharmacol.* 8:491, 1968.

Holzbauer, M., and Vogt. M. *J. Neurochem.* 1:8, 1956.

Huguenard, P. In *Pain*, ed. by A. Soulairac, et al. Academic Press, London, 1968. P. 477.

Ingram, W. R., et al. *Arch. Neurol. Psychiat.* 28:513, 1932.

Janssen, P. A. J. *Int. Rev. Neurobiol.* 8:221, 1965a.

Janssen, P. A. J. *Arzneimittel-Forsch.* (Drug Res.) 15:1196, 1965b.

Janssen, P. A. J. *Int. J. Neuropsychiat.* 3(Suppl. 1):10s, 1967.

Janssen, P. A. J., et al. *Arzneimittel-Forsch.* (Drug Res.) 16:339, 1966.

Janssen, P. A. J., et al. *Arzneimittel-Forsch.* (Drug Res.) 17:841, 1967.

Jouvet, M., In *Psychopharmacology. A Review of Progress*, ed. by D. H. Efron. U.S. Dept. of Health, Education and Welfare, Washington, D.C., 1968. P. 523.

Karczmar, A. G., et al. *Physiol. Behav.* 5:175, 1970.

Killam, E. K. *Pharmacol. Rev.* 14:175, 1962.

Killam, E. K. In *Psychopharmacology. A Review of Progress*, ed. by D. H. Efron. U.S. Dept. of Health, Education and Welfare, Washington, D.C., 1968. P. 411.

Killam, E. K., and Killam, K. F. *J. Pharmacol.* 116:35, 1956.

Kline, N. S. *Ann. N.Y. Acad. Sci.* 59:107, 1954.

Knopp, W. *Int. J. Neuropsychiat.* 3(Suppl. 1):105s, 1967.

Knopp, W., et al. *Current Therap. Res.* 12:115, 1970.

Koella, W. P., et al. *EEG Clin. Neurophysiol.* 25:481, 1968.

Laborit, H., et al. *Presse Méd.* 60:206, 1952.

Longo, V. G. *Electroencephalographic Atlas for Pharmacological Research.* Elsevier, Amsterdam, 1962.

Longo, V. G., and Florio, V. *Acta Psychiat. Belg.* 70:676, 1970.

Longo, V. G., and Napolitano, L. *Il Farmaco* 10:297, 1955.

Longo, V. G. et al. *J. Pharmacol.* 111:49, 1954.

Martin, S. J., et al. *Anesthesiology* 28:458, 1967.

Mellgren, A. *Psychother. Psychosom.* 15:454, 1967.

Miner, R. W., ed. *Reserpine and Other Alkaloids of Rauwolfia Serpentina: Chemistry, Pharmacology, and Clinical Applications.* Ann. N.Y. Acad. Sci. 59:1-140, 1954.

Miner, R. W., ed. *Reserpine in the Treatment of Neuropsychiatric, Neurological and Related Clinical Problems.* Ann. N.Y. Acad. Sci. 61:1-280, 1955.

Morpurgo, C. *Arch. int. Pharmacodyn.* 137:78, 1962.

Morpurgo, C., and Theobald, W. *Psychopharmacologia* 6:178, 1964.

Moruzzi, G., and Magoun, H. W. *EEG Clin. Neurophysiol.* 1:455, 1949.

Munkvad, I., et al. *Brain Behav. Evol.* 1:89, 1968.

Passouant, P., et al. *Compt. Rend. Soc. Biol.* 150:779, 1956.

Pletscher, A., et al. *Science* 122:374, 1955.

Pletscher, A., et al. *Advances in Pharmacol.* 6B:55, 1968.

Plummer, A. J., et al. *Ann. N.Y. Acad. Sci.* 59:8, 1954.

Pscheidt, G. R., et al. *J. Pharmacol.* 144:37, 1964.

Randall, L. O., and Schallek, W. In *Psychopharmacology. A Review of Progress,* ed. by D. H. Efron. U.S. Dept. of Health, Education and Welfare, Washington, D.C., 1968. P. 153.

Rossum, J. M., van In *Neuropsychopharmacology,* ed. by H. Brill. Excerpta Medica Found., Amsterdam, 1967. P. 321.

Schlitter, E., and Plummer, A. J. In *Psychopharmacological Agents,* ed. by M. Gordon. Academic Press, New York, 1964. P. 9.

Schoenheimer, R. *The Dynamic State of Body Constituents.* Harvard University Press, Cambridge, Mass., 1942.

Shepherd, M., et al. *Clinical Psychopharmacology.* English Universities Press, London, 1968.

Sigg, E. B., and Schneider, J. A. *EEG Clin. Neurophysiol.* 2:419, 1957.

Stein, L. and Wise, C. D. *Science* 171:1032, 1971.

Sulser, F., and Bass, A. D. In *Psycopharmacology. A Review of Progress,* ed. by D. H. Efron. U.S. Dept. of Health, Education and Welfare, Washington, D.C., 1968. P. 1065.

CHAPTER 2

Antidepressant Drugs

THE DEPRESSIVE SYNDROME

According to classical concepts, the depressive syndrome (melancholy) constitutes, together with schizophrenia, the group of endogenous psychoses. Melancholy is characterized by affective disturbances, in the sense of lowering (depression) of mood. From the psychiatric viewpoint, there are many ways in which depressions may be classified.

One approach, based on *etiology*, considers three groups:

1. The endogenous depression, which is typified by a phasic course of periods of depression alternating with periods of normality, and in some cases (manic-depressive psychoses) with manic phases (Figure 2.1).

2. The neurotic or reactive depressions, which are relatively benign, consist of an abnormal reaction to stressful events.

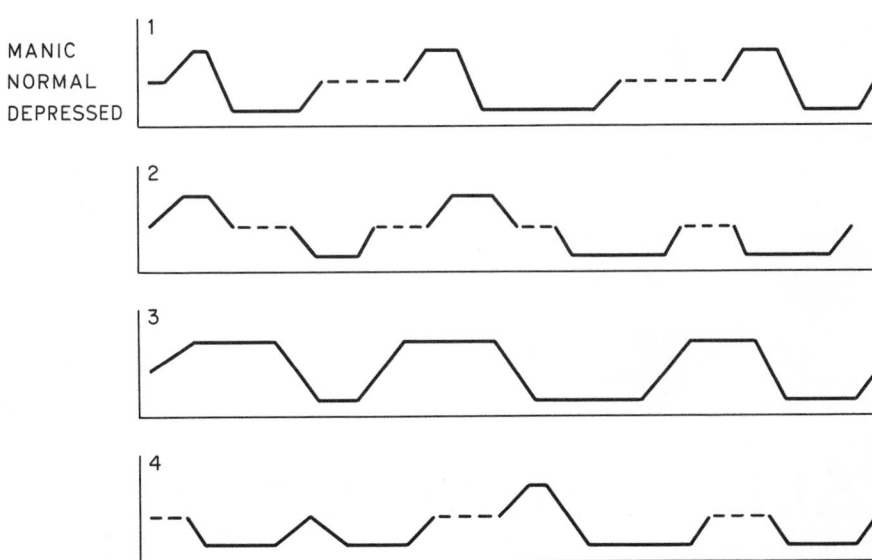

MANIC
NORMAL
DEPRESSED

Figure 2.1
Affective behavior disorders can be either cyclic or sporadic. Some patients show regular alternating recurrences of manic and depressive episodes with or without intervals of normality (schemes **1, 2, 3**). In others, the cyclic disturbances are more irregular, usually with a prevalence of depressive episodes (scheme **4**). More rarely, only depressive or manic episodes can be encountered (redrawn, from Rossini R., Trattato di Psichiatria, Cappelli, Bologna, 1969).

3. The organic depressions, which have an identifiable pathological substrate, appear following degenerative, infective or traumatic processes of the brain.

The basic symptom of depression is a profound, unjustified sadness that can become such a burden for the affected individual that suicide becomes a possibility. At times, instead of a true sadness, the patient shows diminished affective participation in the events and situations that form his environment. Of all the mental disturbances, depression is associated with the highest incidence of attempted or completed suicides. It must also be stressed that a depressed patient, clothed in feelings of complete desperation, may be dangerous to those around him and may be capable of homicide, in an attempt to protect himself or others from threats existing only in his mind. Sadness is often associated with other important symptoms, such as anxiety and anguish, to which must be added somatic and neurovegetative disturbances: insomnia, loss of appetite, diminished libido, polyuria, tachycardia.

The advent of psychopharmacological chemotherapy has made available to the clinician drugs with a specific influence on one or the other of the symptoms (target symptoms) of the depressive syndrome and has given rise to a *phenomenological* subdivision of the various types of depression according to their predominant patterns, that is, retarded depression, anxious depression, inhibited depression, and so forth. Considerable progress has been made in the treatment of depression since this criterion has been accepted by clinicians.

With the introduction of shock-therapy, in the thirties, clinicians finally had in their hands a method of treating depressed patients. The administration of insulin to induce coma, of convulsive therapy with pentamethylentetrazol or electroshock, was the beginning of a new era in psychiatry. Except for amphetamine and barbiturates (in the manic phase), drug therapy at that time was nonexistent, and for this reason shock therapy dominated the field for almost twenty years. Even though this procedure was widely used, many voices were raised against it, not so much on practical grounds, because quite satisfactory results were obtained, but because it was potentially dangerous, distasteful to apply, and above all because of its empiric nature. As a matter of fact, it was difficult to establish any rationale for the treatment, although much work was done to define its mechanism. In the course of this research, it was observed that electroshock was effective in conditions other than mental disturbances (psoriasis, for example). This observation led to a series of hypotheses concerning cerebral humoral alterations that, in the light of present knowledge, seem rather nebulous. Cerletti himself (1950) harbored certain misgivings about his technique, and he repeatedly stated that it would soon be replaced by biochemical treatment. He felt that electroshock, because of its stress on the brain itself, causes the production in the brain of a specific substance, responsible for the therapeutic effect. He attempted to isolate this substance (which he called *acroagonine*) from the brains of pigs subjected to repeated electroshocks, and he treated patients with these extracts, but without success.

In 1957, a series of independent clinical observations reported on the antidepressant effects of two drugs, imipramine and iproniazid, which differed chemically and pharmacologically. With this discovery, depressive syndromes became subject to chemical treatment. It is interesting to note that in this case, as in the initial chemotherapeutic attack on schizophrenia, two distinct drugs were introduced almost concurrently into the clinic.

Iproniazid was first used, along with isoniazid, in the early fifties, in the treatment of tuberculosis (Selikoff et al., 1952); it was noted that in some patients a sense of well-being and mood elevation appeared shortly after the start of therapy, an effect that could not be attributed only to the beneficial effect on the course of the specific process. Additional studies demonstrated that this compound, as well as other hydrazines, inhibits the enzyme monoamine oxidase (MAO) (Zeller, 1952). Eventually, iproniazid was abandoned in the therapy of tuberculosis because of the introduction of more effective compounds; however, it again attracted attention in 1957 when Loomer et al. started to use it as a "psychic energizer" for the treatment of depressed patients.

In the same year, Kuhn reported that encouraging results were obtained with a synthetic developed at the Geigy laboratories, G 22335 (chemically related to chlorpromazine), which underwent clinical trials as an antipsychotic. The clinical observations indicated instead that G 22335, later called imipramine, possessed distinct antidepressive properties. Since that time, numerous compounds belonging to the two categories have been tried in the clinic, and also in the laboratory, where much work was directed toward finding valid screening procedures for the evaluation of compounds with antidepressive properties.

TRICYCLIC ANTIDEPRESSANTS

The first clinical trials with the Geigy derivative G 22355 (imipramine) were done on schizophrenics because the chemical structure of this substance resembled certain phenothiazine derivatives (Figure 2.2). However, the only patients who benefited were those in whom disturbances of mood predominated, particularly negativism, motor retardation, and anxiety. No improvement was noted in the other symptoms of these patients, such as disturbed ideation, hallucinations, and delusions. Encouraged by this favorable outcome, more

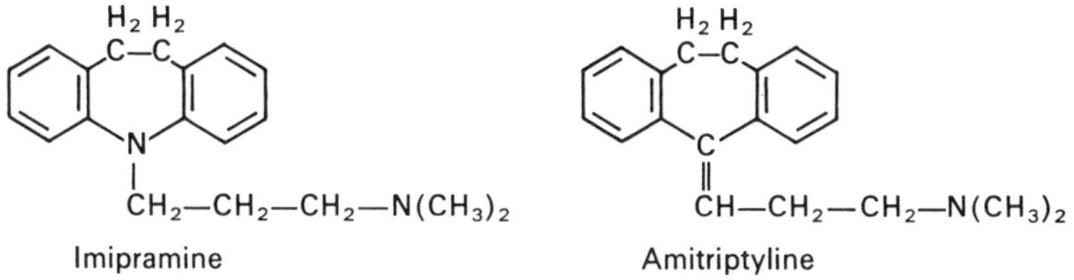

Imipramine

Amitriptyline

Figure 2.2
Chemical structures of **imipramine** and **amitriptyline**. The similarity with the phenothiazines is evident (see Figure 1.2). The imipramine nucleus differs from that of the phenothiazines by the presence of a CH_2—CH_2 bridge instead of an S; that of amitriptyline has, in addition, a C in place of the N. These substances are considered respectively derivatives of imidobenzyl and of cycloheptadiene. For the sake of simplicity and because of their structural formula, they are referred to as "tricyclics."

work was done, both in Europe and America, that confirmed the effectiveness of imipramine in relieving the symptoms of depression. Within a few years, other drugs were introduced into therapy, since many related compounds had already been synthetized and subjected to both laboratory and clinical trials, in which they showed, to varying degrees, anticholinergic, antihistaminic, antiparkinsonian, and sedative properties. In a very short time, the armamentarium of psychiatrists for dealing with depressed patients was enlarged with many products. These can be divided into two groups, which bear some chemical resemblance to each other, in particular, the presence of three rings (hence the name *tricyclic*). These two groups are (*a*) the imidobenzyl derivatives, of which the foremost is imipramine, and (*b*) the derivatives of cycloheptadiene, the prototype of which is amitriptyline (Figure 2.2).

In practice, the therapeutic efficacy of the tricyclic antidepressants is not as pronounced or dependable as that of the antipsychotics. The initial reports regarding the effectiveness of these compounds were not unanimous. This is because the patients who were treated varied tremendously among themselves and, understandably, varied greatly in their response to the drugs. After some experience with these substances, it became apparent that the drugs were effective only upon certain manifestations of the depressive syndrome and that each antidepressant showed itself active against one or another of the aspects of the depressive syndrome. The concept of "target symptom" elaborated by Freyhan (1959) has certainly helped in developing a rationale for the field of antidepressant chemotherapy. At present, therapy varies according to whether the syndrome is predominantly agitated-anxious, retarded-anxious, or inhibited-apathic, and this irrespective of the etiology of the depression (see the preceding section).

Among the tricyclic antidepressants, imipramine is more specific for cases in which mood is depressed; in patients having a high anxiety level, amitriptyline or its analogs seem indicated because of their more marked sedative and anti-anxiety effects. Even though it has been suggested that there is a specific drug for each depressive syndrome, many researchers are not yet convinced of this specificity.

It has been proposed, but not universally accepted, that desipramine is a relatively fast-acting antidepressant. Desipramine differs from the parent imipramine in that it lacks one of the two N-methyl groups. During investigations on the metabolic rate of imipramine in the rat, it was found that the drug was desmethylated, and the delay of its effects was attributed to its transformation into desmethyl-imipramine, which was considered the active compound (Gillette et al., 1961). Desipramine was introduced into the clinic with the claim of a more prompt effect; this effect was not confirmed by controlled trials, which, however, did indicate that disipramine is a good antidepressant.

The clinical effect of antidepressants requires a certain time to become evident, generally a few weeks. This delay has led in the past to an incorrect evaluation of some of these drugs, since in some forms, as for example in the manic-depressive syndrome, the depressive phase tends to remit spontaneously (see Figure 2.1 and comments in the introduction). Therefore, positive results obtained with new antidepressants must be carefully controlled. Keeping in mind that not all patients show beneficial effects from the treatment, in favorable cases, after a week of treatment, the mood-elevating response can be observed. The feelings of grief, self-depreciation and hopelessness attenuate; the patient shows greater animation and becomes less concerned; normal sleep patterns return along with a reduction of the neurovegetative disturbances. The improvement obtained under drug treatment resembles spontaneous remission but takes place more rapidly. Administration of antidepressants must be continued for a long time and must not be discontinued even though the patient has reached a normal state; in fact, if therapy is suspended, the syndrome reappears in its original intensity. It is fortunate that all these compounds are devoid of appreciable chronic toxicity; they can be taken for an extended period without serious inconveniences and without habituation or addiction.

Of the side effects, the more important are the neurovegetative symptoms, which are related to the anticholinergic properties present in various measure in all the tricyclic antidepressants: dryness of the mouth, mydriasis, and dysuria. Extrapyramidal disturbances are practically absent; the fine tremor of the hands and the tongue seen in some patients treated with high doses most likely has some other origin and is similar to that observed in emotional situations. Dangers of the therapy are inherent in the nature of the disease itself. Since the antidepressants often get rid of psychomotor inhibition before influencing other symptoms, patients in this transitional period can be dangerous to others or may attempt suicide.

In many psychiatric centers various methods are used to evaluate the progress of a melancholic patient. These are based on psychomotor tests, tests of intellectual functions, and perceptual tests. Some observations are rather interesting, such as that which regards the appreciation of an apparent horizon, which is lowered in depression. When an antidepressant is given, a raising of the apparent horizon is noticed (Krus et al., 1966). Strangely enough, normal subjects treated with the drug also show the same phenomenon, although they react with sedation to the treatment (Ostfeld, 1961). It should be emphasized that the effect of the antidepressants (as well as that of the antipsychotics) on normal individuals bears little relationship to their therapeutic efficacy. Sedation cannot be equated with antipsychotic effect, nor can stimulation be equated with antidepressive action. In addition to the aforementioned tests, other projections of the psychopathological state of the subject may be available. For example, when depressed patients are encouraged to paint or to draw, they select dark colors and hues, their landscapes are desolate, icy, and without life. With time, as the depression lightens, these patients tend toward a selection of more cheerful subjects, and their scenes become more vivid and full of color. Figure 2.3 shows the amelioration of a psychic depression followed through pictorial expression.

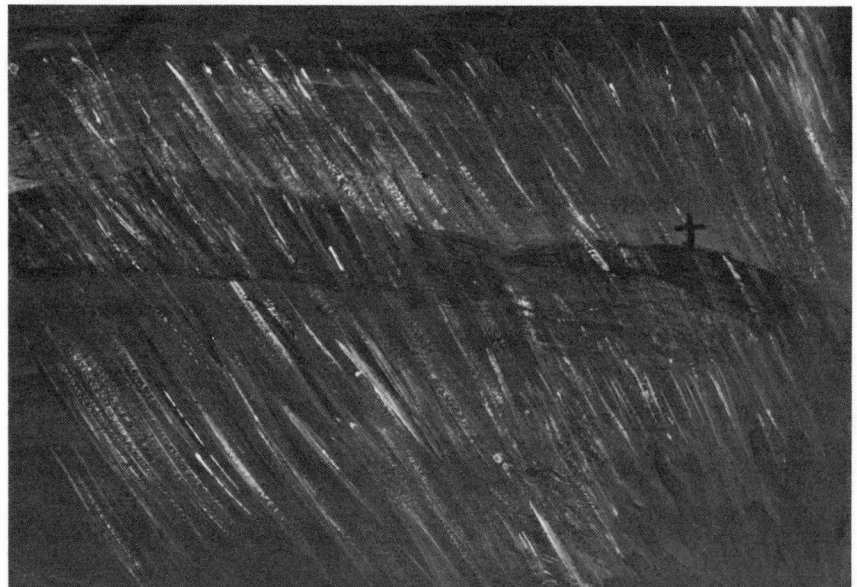

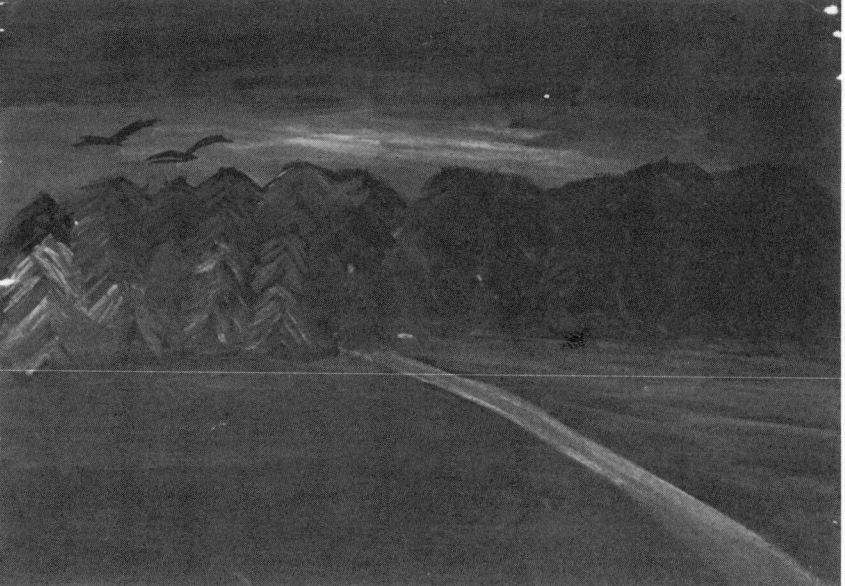

Figure 2.3
Contrary to that observed in schizophrenic and neurotic painters, who create elaborate and imaginative artworks, the production of depressed artists is scarce, because of the prevailing psychomotor inhibition. Some cases exist, in which it has been possible to follow the improvement of the patient through his artistic expression. The first two pictures (*left*), done during a melancholic spell, represent death symbols, black birds, crosses, stormy weather, desolate landscapes without a way of escape. In the other two

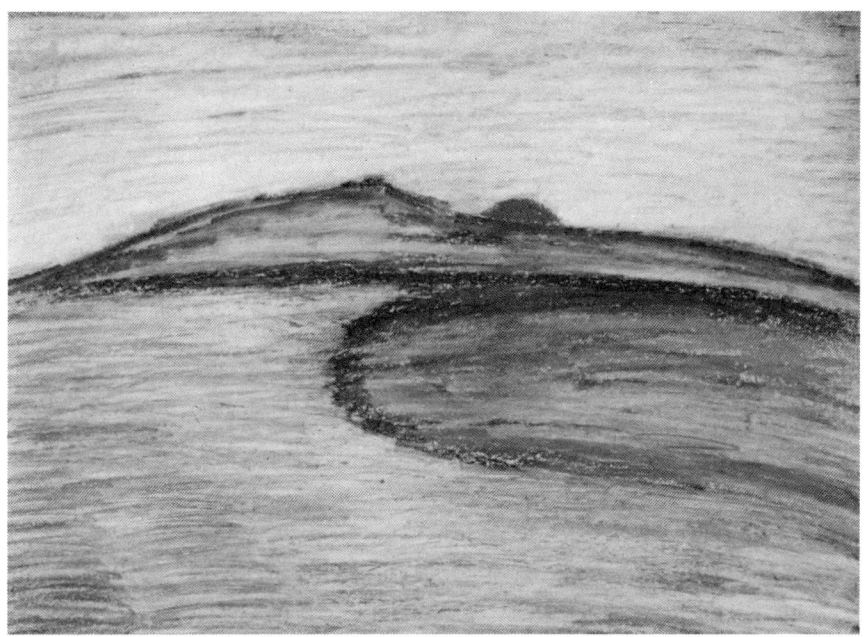

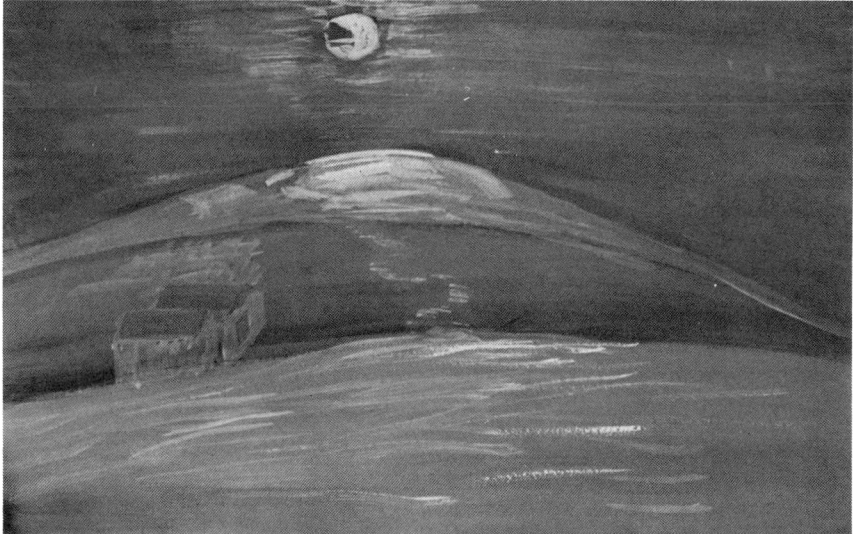

pictures, painted after a cycle of therapy with antidepressants, more movement is depicted, warm tones and colors appear, the houses represent security, and the sunrise reflects hope (from P. Kielholz, *Psicopatologia ed Espressione Figurativa*, vol. 13, Sandoz, 1970).

Effects on Animals

The chemical synthesis of several imidobenzyl derivatives, of which imipramine is one, was reported in 1954 (Schindler and Häfliger), shortly following the pharmacological investigations on chlorpromazine. Initial laboratory studies followed along the same lines as those of the latter, stressing in particular the anticholinergic, antiserotoninergic, and antihistaminic properties of imipramine. It was found also that, at low doses, imipramine possessed no noteworthy effect on motor or conditioned activity. Large doses were followed by motor depression and by reduced spontaneous activity; this effect was similar to that induced by the phenothiazines. After clinical trials in which its antidepressive activity was noted, the drug was again subjected to laboratory evaluation. Imipramine was found to be neither a stimulant nor a MAO inhibitor; it was therefore different from the other antidepressants in current clinical use (iproniazid, the amphetamines). Investigations of peripheral autonomic effects showed, at small doses, an enhancement and prolongation of the vasopressor response to noradrenaline. This latter phenomenon was attributed to a "sensitization" of the adrenergic receptors (Sigg, 1959); by extrapolating these results to the brain Sigg advanced the hypothesis that the antidepressive effect could be due to the sensitization of the cerebral adrenergic synapses.

Research on the central effects of imipramine showed that, in contradistinction to the phenothiazines, the motor depression elicited by imipramine was never accompanied by catatonia. It was also found that imipramine inhibits a number of actions of reserpine and tetrabenazine: palpebral ptosis, diarrhea, sedation, hypothermia, catatonia. The mechanism of this interaction was investigated in detail because the clinical picture observed in man following the administration of reserpine had some points in common with the depressive syndrome (see the discussion of reserpine in Chapter 1). The stimulating and catatonia-relieving actions of imipramine were manifested also in animals treated with other neuroleptics (phenothiazines, butyrophenones), but a peculiar effect was noted in the case of reserpine and tetrabenazine, in that the antagonistic effect was present only if imipramine was administered before reserpine (Sulser et al., 1962). In fact, a "reversal" of the reserpine effect could be elicited: the pretreated animals (rats) showed an increase in spontaneous activity. This phenomenon occurred without blocking the depletion of the cerebral amines caused by reserpine. Many explanations were offered when this phenomenon was described, but some time passed before further experimentation clarified the mechanisms involved.

Research on the kinetics of chemical transmission led to a radical change in the concept of the neurotransmitter liberated at the nerve ending and inactivated locally by more-or-less specific enzymatic processes. It was found, for instance, that the re-utilization (uptake) by the same nerve endings of the liberated mediator or of its metabolites is of primary importance in the regulation of the amount of intra- or extra-neuronal transmitter that is present at a nerve ending. Axelrod et al. (1961), using labeled norepinephrine, demonstrated that imipramine lowers the concentration of this mediator in tissues, while it increases that present in the serum. This suggests that the drug interferes with binding sites, thereby reducing the uptake of norepinephrine from adrenergic terminals (Figure 2.4). By injecting labeled norepinephrine into the lateral ventricles, it was later showed that the same phenomenon (the blockage of uptake) occurred also in the brain (Glowinski and Axelrod, 1964).

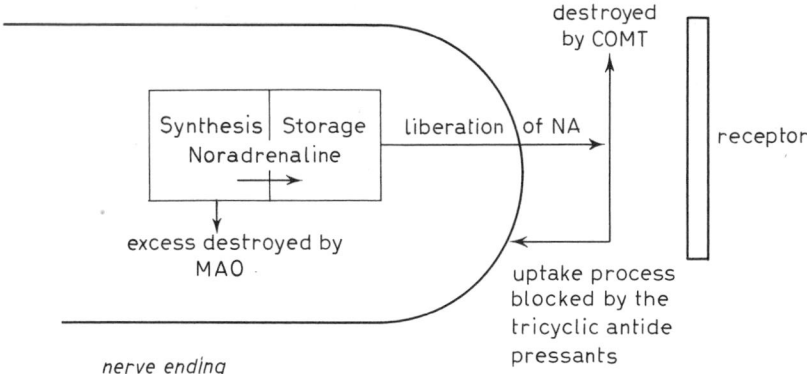

Figure 2.4
Diagram representing the noradrenaline cycle in a sympathetic nerve terminal. Noradrenaline is continuously synthetized and incorporated into storage granules; the excess of the amine is released into the cytoplasm and destroyed by MAO. Upon arrival of the stimulus along the nerve, noradrenaline is liberated into the junction and destroyed by catechol-*o*-methyltransferase (COMT); part of the amine re-enters into the nerve through an active uptake process. The tricyclic antidepressants block this uptake, thus increasing the quantity of the neurohumor outside the nerve endings.

Today, this blockage of uptake of the catecholamines provides the hypothesis that most satisfactorily explains a great part of the effects of the tricyclic antidepressants: (*a*) potentiation, at small doses, of the stimulating effects of the sympathetic nerves on the end organs (attributed by Sigg to a "sensitization"); (*b*) increase in concentration and the persistence of injected norepinephrine in the blood. Also the "reversal" of the effects of reserpine and tetrabenazine can be explained through this mechanism. The administration of tricyclic antidepressants, by inhibiting the uptake of norepinephrine, which is liberated by reserpine, makes available more neurotransmitter at the receptor sites and induces a series of symptoms. In the normal animal these symptoms are very transient or not evident (excitation, hyperthermia, etc.). On the other hand, if the levels of norepinephrine in the brain are already low (some hours after the administration of reserpine for instance), sedation is not reversed by the administration of antidepressants because of the absence of the mediator, the stores of which are depleted by the alkaloid. Similarly, if the catecholamine synthesis is blocked by α-methyl-*p*-tyrosine before the administration of tetrabenazine, the antidepressants no longer antagonize the sedation induced by the drug.

The anticholinergic properties of the tricyclic compounds, already present in imipramine, and even more marked in amitriptyline and its derivatives, attracted the attention of some researchers to the role of this property in their clinical efficacy. Although somewhat atypical, an atropine-like action can be observed in a series of tests involving both peripheral and central receptors (Rathbun and Slater, 1963). Among the centrally-originated effects, those on the EEG and its activation were thoroughly investigated. In rabbits and cats administration of amitriptyline induces after a short delay a synchronization of the EEG waves, which bears a strong similarity to the effect of atropine or scopolamine (Vernier, 1961). Amitriptyline and imipramine proved effective also in antagonizing the EEG patterns of desynchronization induced by various cholinergic agents, such as arecoline, eserine, and nicotine (Rathbun and Slater, 1963; Benesova, 1967). According to some authors, this central atropine-like action is connected with the tranquilizing and anti-anxiety component of the antidepressants, while the adrenomimetic action (depending on the influence on catecholamine uptake) is responsible for the psychomotor stimulation (Benesova, 1970). A central atropine-like action is common to a variety of drugs; only in a few instances can it be linked to calming properties. However, the defect in depression could involve neurotransmitters other than the amines, and a drug that acts both on the adrenergic system and also on the cholinergic system may represent an optimal combination.

Another effect observed in EEG investigations is the inhibition of the appearance of the paradoxical sleep phases in the sequence of the spontaneous sleep. This has been observed both in man and in experimental animals (Rinaldi, 1967). This data can be related to the improvement of enuretic subjects treated with imipramine; it is known, in fact, that bed-wetting occurs during paradoxical sleep periods. This influence on sleep phases could also be of importance in the regularization of the sleep disturbances in depressed patients; abolition of early awakening is one of the first effects observed in the course of antidepressant therapy.

MONOAMINE OXYDASE INHIBITORS

Observations on the euphoric effects of iproniazid date back to 1952 when Selikoff et al. reported that the beneficial effects of this drug were not specifically due to its effect on the basic disease they were studying (tuberculosis) but rather to a psychic reaction on the part of the patient. At the time, this psychological effect was not investigated clinically. However, some work in the laboratory did stir interest in monoamine oxydase inhibitors; this work was directed toward their enzyme-inhibiting properties. The initial stimulus was provided by Zeller (1952), who demonstrated the inhibiting properties of a series of hydrazide derivatives on monoamine oxydase (MAO). MAO is present in many tissues, but especially in liver, brain, heart, ganglia, and the sympathetic nerve endings; it plays an important role in the metabolism of the biogenic amines, converting their terminal amino group to a carbonyl function (Figure 2.5). Its substrates include epinephrine, norepinephrine, serotonin, dopamine, and tyramine. MAO inhibition leads to an increase of these amines and to a reduction of their acid catabolites. Therefore, an influence on these important physiologically active substances would be expected to have far-reaching consequences on body functions, both peripherally and centrally.

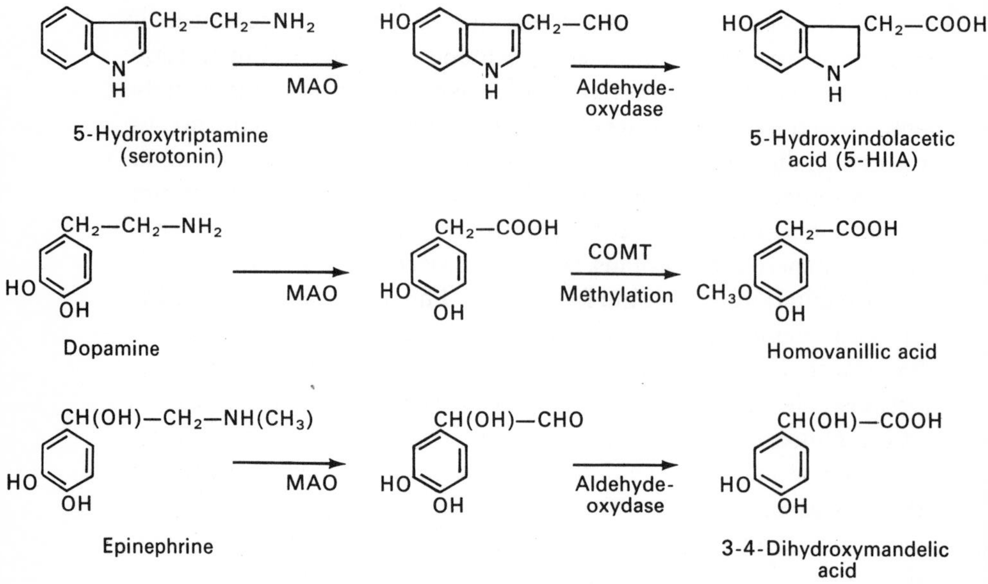

Figure 2.5

Monoamine oxidase (MAO) is responsible for the oxidative deamination of several monoamines of biological interest. The reaction works according to the general equation:

$$R-CH_2-NH_2 + O_2 + H_2O \rightleftarrows R-CHO + NH_3 + H_2O$$

In the scheme are illustrated the routes for the oxidative metabolism of 5-hydroxytriptamine (serotonin), dopamine, and adrenaline (epinephrine). It should be kept in mind that other mechanisms of destruction of the monoamines exist in the body, represented for instance by the catechol-*o*-methyl-transferase (COMT), which methylates the OH group in the ortho position, an example of which is shown in the dopamine degradation (see also Figure 2.4).

Investigations of the properties of MAO inhibitors eventually became associated with the work on neuroleptics. Brodie and Shore (1957) reported that rabbits treated with iproniazid and later injected with reserpine, instead of showing the usual depression, were considerably excited; only a small decline in brain serotonin was found in these animals, which indicated that the released amines had not been metabolized. These observations led to the first theories concerning the role played by serotonin in central transmission; these theories were further elaborated and extended to the other monoamines.

In 1957, Loomer et al. described the antidepressive effect of iproniazid, revealing a new approach for the treatment of melancholy; this report resulted in a vast research effort to develop more effective and less toxic agents. The usual initial enthusiasm related to a new therapeutic lead was such that any drug possessing either *in vitro* or *in vivo* MAO-inhibitory properties was tried in the clinic; unfortunately, some rather severe side effects were encountered and many of the MAO inhibitors have been withdrawn from the market because of their toxic effect. At the present time only a few MAO inhibitors are used clinically (see Figure 2.6).

Concerning the effect in man, a distinction must be made between two groups of drugs. (*a*) The hydrazides and the hydrazines produce their effects only after a certain delay: after a minimum of a week or so, one notes a progressive elevation of mood, a rising sense of joy and optimism. (*b*) Tranylcypromine brings an immediate euphoria and excitement, due probably to the amphetamine moiety of the molecule; this is followed by a steady improvement of mood. Because of this pronounced exciting effect, these substances find their greatest use in retarded depressions. In the most favorable responses there occurs a release of motor inhibition, a reduction in the sense of preoccupation, and increased interaction with the environment. Therapy must be continued for a long period, and, as in the case of the tricyclics, a relapse occurs if it is interrupted.

Side effects are numerous and their incidence high. The excitatory effect implies the same risks as for the tricyclic agents, namely, manic states, suicidal attempts, exteriorization of deliria. Other more specific side effects include orthostatic hypotension, liver damage, and the so-called "cheese reaction," in which patients develop hypertension due to the tyramine content of some fermented cheeses, wines, beers, or yeast extracts. Ingested tyramine, under normal conditions, is inactivated by the liver, but, in the presence of MAO inhibitors, it reaches the general circulation to produce sympathomimetic effects. Other inconveniences are related to the influence of these drugs on other enzymes, and particularly on the liver microsomal oxidative system, which plays an important role in the process of destruction and inactivation of various substances. This inhibition explains the potentiation of the effects and toxicity of sympathomimetics, analgesics, and tricyclic antidepressants.

		Daily dose mg

HYDRAZINES

Phenelzine — C_6H_5—$CH_2CH_2NHNH_2$ — 15-45

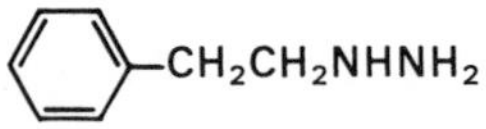

Pheniprazine — C_6H_5—$CH_2CH(CH_3)NHNH_2$ — *not in clinical use*

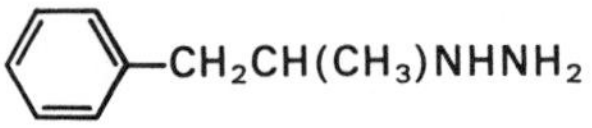

HYDRAZIDES

Iproniazid — (pyridine)—$CONHNHCH(CH_3)_2$ — *not in clinical use*

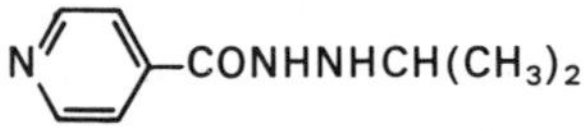

Nialamide — (pyridine)—$CONHNHCH_2CH_2CONHCH_2$—C_6H_5 — 50-200

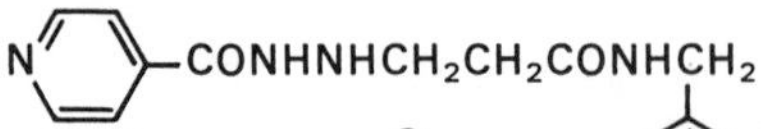

Isocarboxazid — C_6H_5—CH_2NHNHC($=$O)—(isoxazole ring, N-O, CH_3), C_6H_5 — 10-30

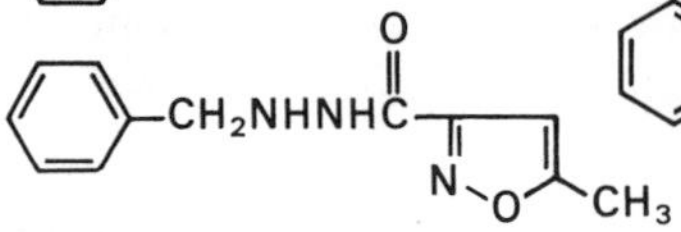

INDOLALKYLAMINES

α-Methyltryptamine — (indole)—$CH_2\overset{CH_3}{\underset{}{C}}HNH_2$ — *not in clinical use*

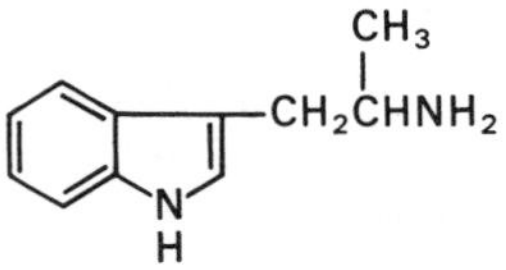

α-Ethyltryptamine — (indole)—$CH_2\overset{C_2H_5}{\underset{}{C}}HNH_2$ — *not in clinical use*

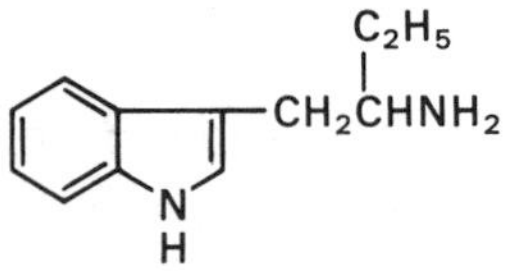

HARMALA ALKALOIDS

Harmine — CH_3O—(β-carboline ring system), N, H, CH_3 — *not in clinical use*

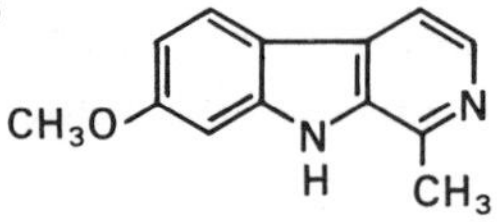

CYCLOPROPYLAMINES

Tranylcypromine — C_6H_5—CH—$CHNH_2$ (cyclopropane, CH_2) — 10-20

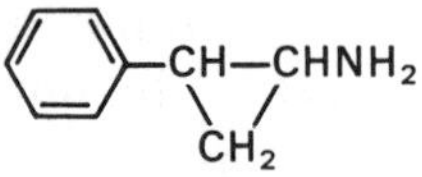

PROPARGYLAMINES

Pargyline — C_6H_5—$CH_2N(CH_3)CH_2C{\equiv}CH$ — 10-50

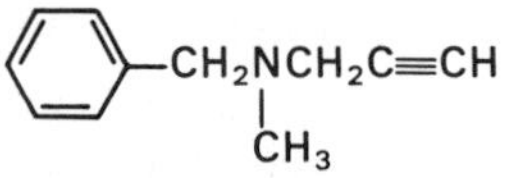

Figure 2.6
Here are the formulas and the generic names of some MAO inhibitors introduced into clinic since 1957. Of these, only five are still in use; the others have been associated with rather serious inconveniences and therefore have been withdrawn from the market. Ethyltryptamine was withdrawn after several cases of agranulocytosis were reported; pheniprazine because of vision disturbances; iproniazid because of the occurrence of hepatic damage. For the effects of harmine see the relevant section of Chapter 4.

In practice, MAO inhibitors should be administered alone; this in part explains their scarce utilization by clinicians, who usually tend to use combined therapy. However, the more important reason of the decline in the clinical use of this class of compounds is that statistics show them to be less efficacious than the tricyclics and electroshock (Bennett, 1967). At present, clinicians tend to reserve use of MAO inhibitors for the uncommon patients refractory to other antidepressive therapies.

MAO inhibitors are used with some success in disease states not psychiatric in nature; for example, pargyline is used in hypertension and in many countries is marketed only with this indication. The hydrazine derivatives are used as adjunctive therapy in anginal syndromes; their mechanism of action in these states has not been clarified. Interestingly, evidence does not necessarily point to improved myocardial irrigation, since subjective improvement occurs without the corresponding ECG changes one would expect.

Laboratory Experimentation with MAO Inhibitors

If one reviews the evolution of the work done on MAO inhibitors since the first observation by Zeller (1952), it becomes apparent that investigations of the mechanism of action of this class of drugs has contributed greatly to the knowledge of the role played by the biogenic amines in the central nervous system. At this point it is extremely instructive to trace the successive steps of this evolution. Zeller's original observations on the action of the various hydrazide derivatives concerned the capability of preventing the *in vitro* oxidation of the bioamines. The first investigative step was therefore to confirm their effects *in vivo* through a series of tests in which MAO inhibitors were administered. These tests measured (*a*) the concentration of various brain amines, which was found to be increased, and (*b*) the urinary excretion of the acid catabolites, which was found to be diminished. The first investigations in man confirmed the diminished urinary excretion of 5-hydroxyindolacetic acid and of 3-methoxy-4-hydroxymandelic acid, which are the main metabolites of indolamines and catecholamines (see Figure 2.5). However, this diminution could be interpreted as a reflection of reduced MAO activity at the periphery that would not necessarily be asso-

ciated with a central effect. Later, autopsy studies indicated that
the MAO inhibitors increase brain amines in the human cerebrum
(Ganrot et al., 1962). Along these lines, it should be mentioned that
some studies performed on amine contents of brains of people who
committed suicide showed, in some cases, a reduction of serotonin
(Shaw et al., 1967) or of its metabolite 5-hydroxyindolacetic acid
(Bourne et al., 1968). For apparent reasons, only limited data are
available, and these observations require confirmation.

Several investigations have been devoted to the study of correlations between behavioral effects and the increase in brain neurotransmitters. In this area, many difficulties were encountered. First
of all, some of the pharmacological effects of the MAO inhibitors
are independent of their enzyme-inhibiting properties; this is particularly true for those derivatives, such as pheniprazine and tranylcypromine, containing in their structures the phenylethylamine
moiety, which confers amphetamine-like properties to these substances. These drugs give rise almost immediately to behavioral
stimulation that is not connected with MAO inhibition; the latter
requires a much longer period of time to develop. However, by
using MAO inhibitors devoid of direct stimulating effects and by
controlling doses and times of administration, it was possible to demonstrate an increase in spontaneous activity with a slow onset and a
prolonged duration. Another difficulty arose when attempts were
made to interpret the latter results in terms of brain-amine content.
Since the inhibition caused by these substances is irreversible, it was
expected that there would be a progressive increase of central and
peripheral indolamine and catecholamine content. It was found
instead that the kinetics of this increase differ with the various
products and are different for the two principal amines considered
(Figure 2.7). In addition, in some animals, for instance the cat and
the dog, serotonin increases and noradrenaline levels remain unaffected (Spector et al., 1960). All these data indicated that any
oversimplified interpretation in such a complex subject as catecholamines and serotonin metabolism must be viewed with caution. A
large step forward occurred when the concept emerged that the
main role of MAO, at least in the brain, is an intracellular one (see
Figure 2.4). MAO is said to regulate amine levels *within* the nerve
endings. In this way, the levels of the amines would be automatically

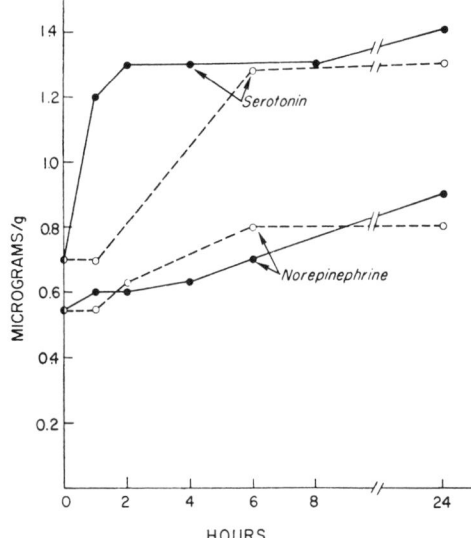

Figure 2.7
The rate of increase of different brain amines varies with the type of MAO inhibitor. The diagram shows the increase in brain serotonin and norepinephrine after administration of iproniazid (*broken lines*) and pheniprazine (*solid lines*) to the rabbit. Each value represents the average of 3 to 5 animals treated respectively with 100 mg/kg of iproniazid and 2 mg/kg of pheniprazine (from Spector et al., 1960. © The Williams & Wilkins Co., Baltimore.)

limited by their excess, which inhibits the process of synthesis. Moreover, in the organism, there are other catabolic pathways that are activated or potentiated in emergency states; therefore, these increases in amines are maintained within relatively restricted limits.

At any rate, it is possible to demonstrate a potentiation both of the behavioral effects of serotonin precursors (5-hydroxytryptophan, tryptamine) and of the catecholamine precursors (DOPA). The test proposed by Tedeschi et al. (1959) employs small doses of tryptamine that, when administered to the rat, cause transient tremors; following treatment with MAO inhibitors, these tremors become more intense and last longer. The test used by Everett and Wiegand (1962) concerns the increase of the behavioral response of mice to DOPA. In animals pretreated with MAO inhibitors, the DOPA challenge results in a marked enhancement of the effects of DOPA, with squeaking, jumping, fighting, and catatonic postures. Both of these tests are widely used for the evaluation of MAO-inhibiting drugs, together with a test that concerns the antagonism or the "reversal" of reserpine or tetrabenazine effects, already described for the tricyclic antidepressants (see page 56).

Depression is perhaps the only syndrome that can be spontaneously observed in some animals without resorting to experimental manipulations (such as the operant-conditioning techniques mentioned in Chapter 1). We know that after the loss of their mate or master some animals develop symptoms that bear a certain similarity to those observed in reactive depressions in man. But immense difficulties are involved in testing antidepressants in these animals; these difficulties explain the lack of data on this subject.

Among experimental psychological studies, those concerning the technique of self-stimulation developed by Olds and Milner (1954) are worth mentioning. In these studies, rats may press a lever to deliver an electric shock to their own brain through implanted electrodes. When the electrodes are located in the lateral or posterior hypothalamus, limbic system, or mesencephalic tegmentum, the rats will repetitively induce brain stimulation. From this finding it was hypothesized that a neuronal system for reward (or pleasure?) exists in the brain; a possible relation of this system to human affective experience has been suggested (Stein, 1962). Stein assumes that in depressed patients the brain centers for positive reinforcement (reward) are hypoactive, and drugs effective against depression probably increase the ability of the brain to respond to positive reinforcement. The results obtained using this technique would indicate that the catecholamines serve excitatory functions in the reward system. Stimulants such as amphetamine increase the rate of stimulation. Imipramine alone is without appreciable effect, but it potentiates the enhancing effect of amphetamine (Stein, 1962). On the other hand, MAO inhibitors at doses that do not influence spontaneous motor activity do exert excitatory effects on self-stimulation and reverse the effects of tetrabenazine on performance (Poschel and Ninteman, 1963, 1964) (Figure 2.8).

In addition to the effects related to MAO inhibition, there are other effects of MAO inhibitors, which are possibly of a different origin. The antianginal and antihypertensive properties of these drugs have been noted only in man, and all attempts to determine these effects in the experimental animal and to correlate them to biochemical data have led to controversial results. According to Schoepke and Wiegand (1963), there is no relationship between changes in myocardial and ganglionic noradrenaline and the lowering of blood pressure observed after pargyline. A number of hydra-

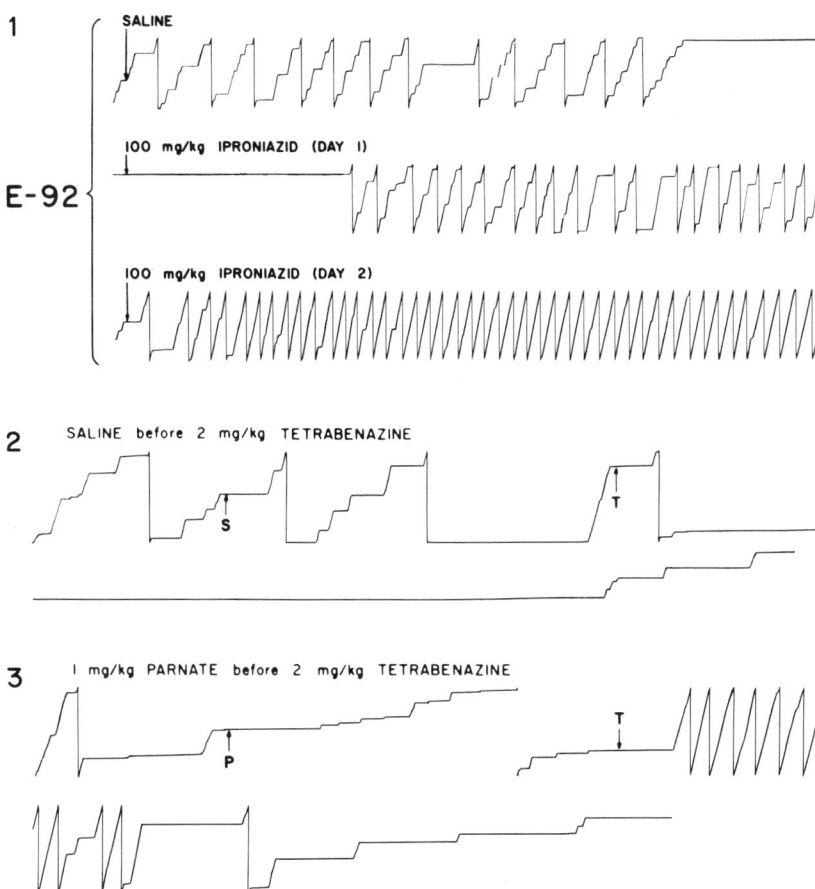

Figure 2.8
Cumulative records of self-stimulation from rats implanted with permanent electrodes in the postero-lateral hypothalamus. Records are 4½ hours long; each reset of the recorder pen equals 550 stimulations. **(1)** The upper series of tracings illustrates the effect of iproniazid. The animal's performance is not modified after saline injection; iproniazid does not have a strong effect until the second day of treatment. The general behavior of the rat is not visibly altered by the drug; therefore, the increase in self-stimulation has been attributed to an increase in the excitability of the reward system. In records **(2)** and **(3)**, the "reversal" of the depressant effects of tetrabenazine by means of pretreatment with tranylcypromine is illustrated. Injection of saline **(S)** does not affect the negative influence of tetrabenazine **(T)** on self-stimulation; on the other hand, the performance increases sharply following the administration of tetrabenazine after pretreatment with tranylcypromine (Parnate) at doses that *per se* have no effect on self-stimulation. All drugs are administered intraperitoneally. (From Poschel and Ninteman, 1963 and 1964).

zine derivatives antagonize pentamethylentetrazol seizures, and this activity seems to correspond to the increase in brain amine levels, although some authors (Balzar et al., 1961) suggest that γ-amino-butyric acid (GABA) might be involved in the anticonvulsant effect. The influence of these compounds on the effects of various drugs was first noticed in the clinic; it practically prevents any combined administration of MAO inhibitors with other drugs. This influence has been investigated and confirmed experimentally. There is a potentiation of barbiturates, narcotics, antipyretics, and amphetamine, and this appears to be dependent upon an effect on a "drug detoxifying enzyme" at the microsomal level, sensitive to these drugs with dose-response and time-effect relationships completely different from those for MAO enzymes.

Investigations of antidepressant drugs have greatly aided those seeking to understand the mechanism of humoral transmission. On the one hand, MAO inhibitors revealed the pathways of monoamine synthesis and destruction; on the other, the tricyclic antidepressants have helped to clarify the process that regulates the levels of monoamines in circulation and residing in local tissue. This process is the uptake of the liberated neurotransmitters by nerve terminals. These two mechanism of action are not widely separated or independent. In fact, it is highly probable that there is a very close link between the intraneuronal presence of the neurotransmitter (influenced by MAO inhibitors) and the extraneuronal content (influenced by the uptake inhibitors). The various bioamines should not be considered only as transmitters, but also as modulators. this second role being as important as the first one. The role of the transmitter is tied to the arrival of the nerve impulse, to the mass liberation of the substance, and to the response of the receptor; the role of the modulator regulates the intraneuronal and extraneuronal presence of the substance and probably conditions the sensitivity of the receptor, the synthesis, and the liberation of the substance and of other neurotransmitters. Within this frame of reference, the theory of Hendley and Snyder (1968) should be mentioned. The theory, which is supported by some experimental results, points to an influence of MAO inhibitors on the uptake of catecholamines. These findings raise the possibility that there may be a unitary explanation of the mode of action of the two classes of antidepressants.

LITHIUM

Lithium, like sodium and potassium, belongs to the chemical group called the alkali metals. Historically, lithium can be considered the first psychotropic drug introduced into Western medicine for the treatment of mental diseases. Back in 1949, the first report of Cade, an Australian physician, was published, concerning the beneficial therapeutic effect of lithium in manic patients. The clinical trials grew out of laboratory research in which Cade had noticed a calming action of lithium salts on animals. However, this action was obtained with very high doses and therefore could be attributed to a toxic effect. Furthermore, the time required to obtain the therapeutic effects and the irregularity with which manic states occur justified the skepticism that arose concerning this form of treatment.

With the advent of the chemotherapy of the depressive syndrome, renewed interest centered upon Cade's work. Danish authors (see Schou, 1963) confirmed with controlled experiments the efficacy of lithium in preventing the appearance of the manic phases in manic-depressive psychoses. (Generally, 250 mg of lithium carbonate three times a day is sufficient although higher doses may be used.) This effect was of great interest because, though various tricyclics and MAO inhibitors were effective in the depressive phase, manic episodes were still treated therapeutically by electroshock. The neuroleptics were in fact found to be without a specific action on the derangement of mood and were able to control the periods of elation and hyperactivity only at high doses that also affected mental processes.

Experimental work with lithium has been particularly poor in results; in fact, no clear-cut pharmacological effect of the substance has yet been demonstrated. There are some biochemical data, however, that suggest an influence on amine metabolism in the opposite direction from that produced by the tricyclic antidepressants, in the sense that lithium either increases the uptake or decreases the release of biogenic amines (Davis, 1970). The results of Matussek and Linsmayer (1968) can be interpreted along these lines; these authors demonstrated that in rats lithium prevents the hyperactivity induced by a combination of desipramine and RO 4-1254, a reserpine-like drug (see page 56).

Another explanation has been advanced in the case of lithium, correlated with its action on the electrolytic balance. This aspect has been investigated extensively, but consistent results have not been reached because ionic balance and water balance are affected by many variables. Some observations, however, point to a decrease of total body water or extracellular fluid during the depressive periods.

In conclusion, many of the results obtained in the laboratory and the clinic indicate that an alteration of the quantity and distribution of brain amines may underlie manic-depressive states. Table 2.1,

Table 2.1 *Effects of Drugs on Amines and Depression*

Drug	Action	Result
Tricyclic antidepressants	Block uptake of norepinephrine (NE) and 5-hydroxy-tryptamine (5-HT)	Relieve depression
MAO inhibitors	Elevate brain levels of NE and 5-HT	Relieve depression
Electroshock	Increases turnover of NE	Relieves depression
Lithium	Increases net uptake of NE and 5-HT, and reduces nerve-stimulated release of NE and 5-HT	Relieves mania
Methysergide	Tryptamine antagonist	Relieves mania
Reserpine	Depletes brain of NE and 5-HT	Causes depression
Propranolol	β-Adrenergic blocker	Causes depression

borrowed from Davis (1970), contains the data that are relevant to this theory. In this table there is some material that has not been discussed, regarding propanolol, methysergide, and biochemical effects of electroshock. All these data provide new leads for research on depressed states, which still present many problems requiring further elucidation.

References

Axelrod, J., et al. *Science* 133:383, 1961.

Balzer, H., et al. *Experientia* 17:38, 1961.

Benesova, O. In *Antidepressant Drugs*, ed. by S. Garattini and M. N. G. Dukes. Excerpta Medica Found., Amsterdam, 1967. P. 247.

Benesova, O. *Activ. Nerv. Super.* 12:226, 1970.

Bennett, I. F. In *Antidepressant Drugs*, ed. by S. Garattini and M. N. G. Dukes. Excerpta Medica Found., Amsterdam, 1967. P. 375.

Bourne, H. R., et al. *Lancet*, ii:805, 1968.

Brodie, B. B., and Shore, P. A. *Ann. N.Y. Acad. Sci.* 66:631, 1957.

Cade, J. F. J. *Med. J. Aust.* 2:349, 1949.

Cerletti, U. *Rapports du Congrès International de Psychiatrie*, Paris, 4:1, 1950.

Davis, J. M. *Int. Rev. Neurobiol.* 12:145, 1970.

Everett, G. M., and Wiegand, R. G. *Biochem. Pharmacol.* 8:85, 1962.

Freyhan, F. A. *Can. Psychiat. Assoc. J.* 4:86, 1959.

Ganrot, P. O., et al. *Experientia* 18:260, 1962.

Gillette, J. R., et al. *Experientia* 17:417, 1961.

Glowinski, J., and Axelrod, J. *Nature* 204:1318, 1964.

Hendley, E. D., and Snyder, S. H. *Nature* 220:1330, 1968.

Krus, D. M., et al. *Arch. Gen. Psychiat.* 14:419, 1966.

Kuhn, R. *Schweiz. Med. Wochenschr.* 87:1135, 1957.

Loomer, H. P., et al. *Psychiat. Res. Rep. Amer. Psychiat. Assoc.* 8:129, 1957.

Matussek, N. and Linsmayer, M. *Life Sci.* 7 (Part 1):371, 1968.

Olds, J. and Milner, P. *J. Comp. Physiol. Psychol.* 47:419, 1954.

Ostfeld, A. M. *Dis. Nerv. Syst.* 22 (Suppl.):24, 1961.

Poschel, B. P. H., and Ninteman, F. W. *Life Sci.* 2:782, 1963.

Poschel, B. P. H., and Ninteman, F. W. *Life Sci.* 3:903, 1964.

Rathbun, R. C., and Slater, I. H. *Psychopharmacologia* 4:114, 1963.

Rinaldi, F. In *Antidepressant Drugs,* ed. by S. Garattini and M. N. G. Dukes. Excerpta Medica Found., Amsterdam, 1967. P. 99.

Schindler, W., and Häfliger, F. *Helv. Chim. Acta* 37:472, 1954.

Schoepke, H. G., and Wiegand, R. G. *Ann. N.Y. Acad. Sci.* 107:924, 1963.

Selikoff, I., et al. *J. Amer. Med. Assoc.* 150:973, 1952.

Schou, M. *Brit. J. Psychiat.* 109:803, 1963.

Sigg, E. B. *Can. Psychiat. Assoc. J.* 4:S75, 1959.

Shaw, D. M. *Brit. J. Psychiat.* 113:1407, 1967.

Spector, S., et al. *J. Pharmacol.* 128:15, 1960.

Stein, L. In *First Hanneman Symposium on Psychosomatic Medicine,* ed. by J. H. Nodine and J. H. Moyer. Lea & Febiger, Philadelphia, 1962. P. 297.

Sulser, F., et al. *Ann. N.Y. Acad. Sci.* 96:279, 1962.

Tedeschi, D. H., et al. *J. Pharmacol.* 126:223, 1959.

Vernier, V. G. *Dis. Nerv. Syst.* 22 (Suppl.):7, 1961.

Zeller, E. A. *Experientia* 8:349, 1952.

CHAPTER 3

Tranquilizing Drugs

MEPROBAMATE AND RELATED DRUGS

It will be recalled from the introductory section that it is now possible, because of the vast amount of clinical experience, to classify the various drugs used in neuropsychiatry according to the mental disorders they affect. Distinct from the psychoses, and particularly from schizophrenia, there exists a large spectrum of psychic disturbances called *neuroses,* which are characterized by anxiety, tension, mild depression, and other emotional disturbances. The drugs of the phenothiazine group, employed successfully in many forms of psychoses, have also been used in the treatment of neuroses. It was observed that phenothiazines, given in moderate dosages, favorably influenced agitation and tension; however, patients with neurotic depression, hypochondriasis, and hysterical symptoms responded poorly.

In the period immediately preceding the "discovery" of anti-psychotic drugs, laboratory studies were conducted on a series of glycerol ethers that possessed the ability to cause hypotonia and muscular paralysis through a central mechanism. Berger (1947), in particular, described the pharmacological properties of *o*-toluoloxy-propanediol (mephenesin). This led to the clinical testing of the drug in some neurological diseases such as spastic states, athetosis, parkinsonism, and as an adjuvant in anesthesia, to obtain muscle relaxation (Berger and Schwartz, 1948). The results were not very encouraging; in neurological syndromes, a positive result often was obtained but the short duration of action hindered its practical application; in anesthetic practice, the administration of concentrated solutions intravenously was responsible for a series of dangerous reactions, both local (thrombosis) and systemic (ematuria). In the course of these trials, it was noted that some of the patients became calm and sedated following drug administration; this response was of the same transitory nature as the other somatic effects. This observation, however, stimulated laboratory attempts to modify the mephenesin molecule so as to obtain more effective drugs.

Meprobamate, the First Tranquilizer

Among the various compounds studied in the laboratory, an aliphatic derivative 2-methyl-2-*n*-proply-1-3-propanediol dicarbamate, or meprobamate (Berger, 1954), demonstrated a long-lasting paralyzing effect, although on a dosage basis it was not more active than mephenesin. The first clinical results with meprobamate were published in 1955 (Selling) and the drug enjoyed rapid and wide acceptance in the treatment of various psychoneurotic states. Today there is a tendency to reappraise the therapeutic value of meprobamate, and much criticism has been showered upon the methods with which it had been originally evaluated (Domino, 1962); however, many favorable reports were published in the early years of its clinical application, regarding its effectiveness in conditions in which anxiety and tension were prominent factors. The effect of meprobamate on psychoneurotic patients was often described as tranquilizing and relaxing. The drug was considered very useful in initiating feelings of improvement and cooperation in psychotherapeutic practices. Also, good results were obtained in the treatment of states of anxiety and angry resentment in the course of alcohol withdrawal. On the other hand, the drug was found to be of little help in psychoses, manic excitement, and in the psychic symptoms of cerebral arteriosclerosis.

The success of meprobamate was in part due to the advantages the drug had over barbiturates, which had been used in the treatment of neuroses. In clinical trials involving both meprobamate and barbiturates, an interesting observation was made, regarding the anxiolitic effect. It was noted that the beneficial influence on the neurotic symptoms was not dependent upon a hypnotic-sedative action but rather was related to the myorelaxant effect. Both the barbiturates and the meprobamate had this effect, but in the latter it appeared at dosages not affecting motor or intellectual performances. Strange as it may seem, there is a rather strict relationship between the myorelaxant properties and the beneficial effect on anxiety and tension. Further on in this chapter, experimental data concerning the origin of this effect will be discussed, however, from the clinical viewpoint, this topic will be dealt with in the light of the current concepts of psychosomatic medicine. It is well known that the clinical picture of anxiety states varies among individuals. In addition to the psychic symptoms, in some patients muscular tension and motor excitement prevail, while in others the neurovegetative disturbances are dominant, involving chiefly the cardiovascular and gastrointestinal systems. The complex alterations of the anxiety state are due according to some authors (see Gellhorn, 1965) to the hyperactivity of the so-called central ergotropic system. The excessive discharge of the ergotropic system, located in the hypothalamus, is thought to be responsible both for the somatic and neurovegetative symptoms observed in neuroses.

A therapy of "progressive relaxation" was developed that, in some cases, helped neurotic patients (Jacobson, 1938). This form of therapy was based on the assumption that a decrease in muscle tension, diminishing the proprioceptive feedback to the centers, would lessen the excitation of the ergotropic system, thereby exerting a beneficial influence on all the components of the anxiety syndrome. (A drug that diminishes muscular tension would presumably act through the same mechanism, with the advantage that relaxation is obtained without the complex training connected with the progressive-relaxation procedure.)

Following in the wake of the tremendous success obtained by meprobamate, many drugs were introduced in the clinic in the course of few years; they were selected by pharmacological screening that showed them to have central paralyzing properties. Some of these (see Figure 3.1), such as carisoprodol, tybamate, and mebutamate can be considered derivatives of meprobamate; others (see Figure 3.2) are chemically different and include zoxazolamine, phenaglycodol, and phenyramidol. None of these drugs proved more effective than meprobamate in treating anxiety states, even though some of them demonstrated other effects, such as pain-killing (carisoprodol, phenyramidol) or antihypertensive actions (mebutamate).

The doses of meprobamate used in the treatment of psychoneurotic patients average between 1200 and 1600 mg per day, distributed in three to four administrations. For the other derivatives

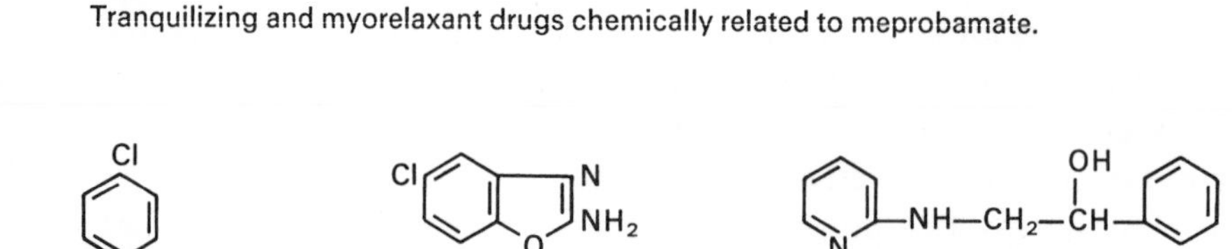

Figure 3.1
Tranquilizing and myorelaxant drugs chemically related to meprobamate.

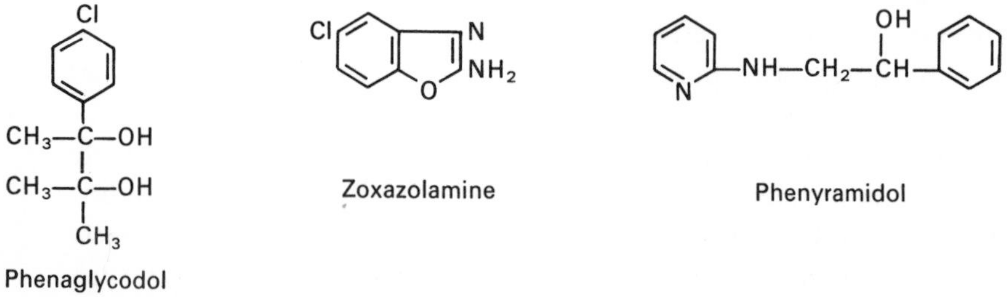

Figure 3.2
Other myorelaxant drugs employed in the clinic as tranquilizers.

(tybamate, mebutamate) the doses are slightly lower. In addition to the psychiatric conditions, it should be recalled that these substances are used in various orthopedic, rheumatic, and neurological diseases, where increased muscle tension is a factor. Meprobamate was also found to be of considerable value for the induction of sleep, probably through its beneficial influence on anxiety and tension that prevent its natural onset.

Side effects with meprobamate occur rarely; some patients complain of drowsiness and cases of allergic reactions have been reported. Administration of meprobamate for prolonged periods of time leads to tolerance and to physical dependence. Abrupt withdrawal produces many of the same signs of abstinence that are observed with barbiturates (tremors, ataxia, hallucinations, anxiety, and in some instances *grand mal* seizures). It seems however that dependence to meprobamate and serious withdrawal disturbances appear only following very high doses (3.5 g per day).

The Effects of Meprobamate and Other Myorelaxant Drugs on Animals

The first description in animals of the paralysis due to drugs having a centrally-mediated myorelaxant effect is probably that of Gilbert and Descomps (1910) for phenoxypropanediol. This compound belonged to a series synthetized by Fourneau, and its paralyzing action was considered only a side effect. The drug was subsequently introduced into therapy as an analgesic and antipyretic under the name of Antodyne. More than thirty years passed before laboratory work was again done on myorelaxants of this type. Goodman et al. in 1943 described this activity for benzimidazole and Berger and Bradley (1946) reported in detail the mechanism of the paralysis produced by ortotoluoloxypropanediol (mephenesin). The toxic syndrome produced by mephenesin in laboratory animals can be described as an ascending paralysis. One first notes hypotonia and then relaxation of the limb muscles; the respiratory muscles are affected with high doses (around 150 mg/kg, intravenous) and death ensues because of asphyxia. The sensorium is not noticeably altered by doses causing paralysis, and neuromuscular transmission remains unchanged. On the other hand, using appropriate tech-

niques, it is possible to demonstrate a depressing effect of mephenesin on some spinal reflexes. Berger (1947) found that the crossed
extension and the flexor reflexes (both polysynaptic) were abolished
by subparalytic doses of mephenesin and that the patellar reflex
(kneejerk) was unaltered. This was subsequently confirmed with
the electrophysiological techniques (by registering the action potentials at the anterior roots following stimulation of an afferent
nerve or of the posterior roots). On the basis of latencies, the mixed
segmental reflex can be divided into a monosynaptic potential
(latency 1–2 msec), representing impulses traversing a single
synapse, and a number of polysynaptic potentials (between 5–40
msec) representing discharges mediated through more complex
arcs, involving several interneurons. The patellar reflex is monosynaptic while the flexor and the crossed extension reflexes are polysynaptic. Accordingly, mephenesin eliminates the polysynaptic
potentials without affecting the monosynaptic (Figure 3.3). Further

Figure 3.3
Effect of mephenesin on the monosynaptic and polysynaptic spinal
cord reflexes in the cat *encéphale
isolé*. The segmental reflex potentials were recorded from the S_1
ventral root; the corresponding dorsal root was stimulated with single
shocks. The first spike, representing
the discharge of monosynaptic arc,
remained unaltered in the course of
the treatment; the potentials due to
the asynchronous discharge of the
interneurons were depressed by the
intravenous administration of 30
and 60 mg/kg of the drug.

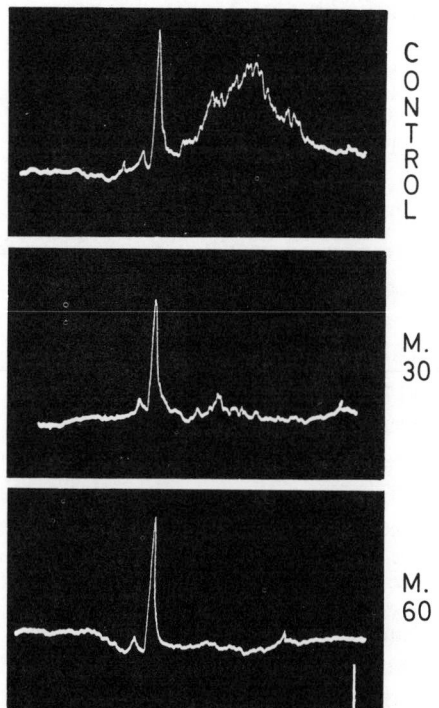

C
O
N
T
R
O
L

M.
30

M.
60

investigations showed that this depressing action on the polysynaptic chains was not limited to the spinal cord but extended rostrally, involving, for example, the linguo-mandibular reflex (King and Unna, 1954). The cortical, diencephalic, and mesencephalic areas responsible for facilitation and inhibition of motor reflexes are also influenced by mephenesin. The patellar reflex can be facilitated or inhibited by electrical stimulation of some higher centers. Facilitation is obtained, for instance, with stimulation of the hypothalamus, while inhibition results from stimulation of the lower pons or of the caudate nucleus. Mephenesin decreases or abolishes facilitatory and inhibitory impulses reaching anterior horn motoneurons from all levels of the brain (Figure 3.4); smaller doses are required to eliminate the influence of the more rostral parts than those of the more caudal parts (Kaada, 1950).

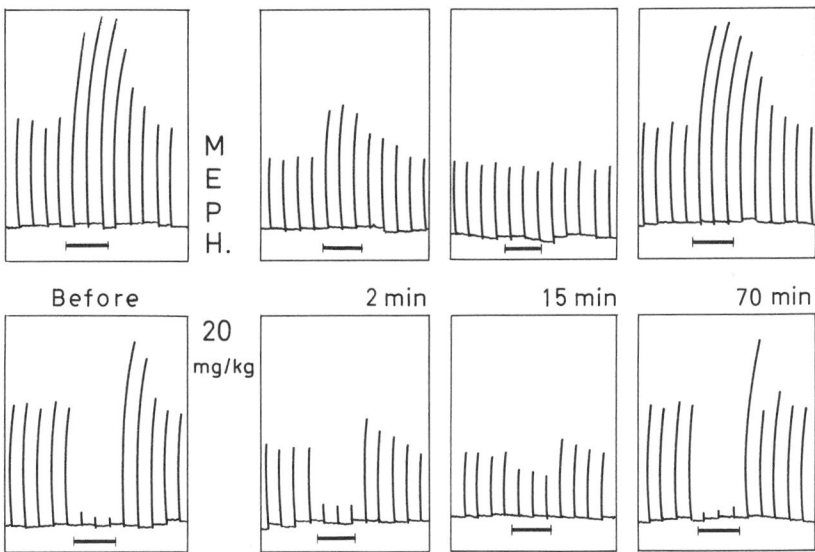

Figure 3.4
Effects of mephenesin on facilitation and inhibition of patellar reflex due to the electrical stimulation of different areas of the brainstem recticular formation. Records of knee jerks elicited by mechanical tapping of the quadriceps tendon every five seconds in a cat under chloralose anesthesia. The *upper line* shows facilitation of the response during stimulation of the pontine region; the *lower line* shows inhibition during stimulation of the bulbar region. After mephenesin, some inhibitory effect is still present, while facilitation is abolished. (Redrawn, from Kaada, 1950.)

Figure 3.5
An unconventional model of the spasticity due to decerebration is given in
the booklet of Magoun and Rhines
(1947) on spasticity. The mechanism
leading to the exaggeration of the
postural reflexes resembles that of a
jack-in-the-box. Jack's hyperactivity
depends both on removal of the lid that
holds him down (supraspinal influences) and on the spring that
pushes him up (spinal reflex arc). (From
Spasticity and the Stretch Reflex, 1947.
Courtesy of Charles C. Thomas, Pub-
lisher, Springfield, Illinois.)

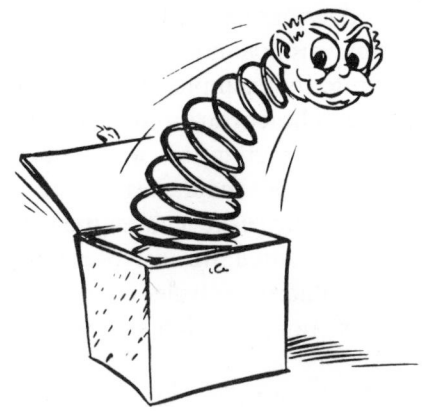

Since the initial studies demonstrated a depressing action on
spinal reflexes, mephenesin was defined as a "spinal-cord depressant"
(Berger, 1949). The term "interneuronic blocking agent" was suggested when further investigations showed an inhibiting action on
the central transmission mediated by interneurons throughout the
entire cerebrospinal axis. Some actions of mephenesin can be considered to be a direct consequence of this effect, for example, the
antagonism to strychnine-induced convulsions or the lytic action on
various spastic states of central origin, such as decerebrate rigidity.
Section of the cerebrum from the midcollicular line to the rostral
edge of the pons elicits in the animal a spastic state due to a disequilibrium in the postural integration. The reflex arc for posture and
muscle tonicity is regulated at the spinal level by proprioceptive impulses deriving from limb muscles, involving the so-called gamma
motor system, innervating the muscle spindles. A midcollicular section of the cerebrum eliminates a great part of the inhibitory influences on this segmental reflex, thus provoking an exaggeration of the
postural reflexes, leading to rigidity and hyperreflexia (Figure 3.5).
The relieving effects of mephenesin on the spasticity and hyperreflexia of the decerebrate animal is mainly due to an influence at the
segmental level, blocking the conduction through the interneurons
subserving the stretch reflex. The possibility cannot be excluded,
however, that a reduction of rigidity is due to more rostral influences, through an action on the supraspinal facilitatory centers.

Aside from these central effects, mephenesin does not have any significant action on other organs and systems. This is quite interesting when one considers that other drugs show various central and peripheral actions, which in some instances interfere with clinical uses.

The effects of mephenesin have been described in detail because it is a prototype of the myorelaxant drugs, including meprobamate. The effects of these drugs on laboratory animals may be summarized as follows—

1. Loss of muscle tone at small doses and paralysis at high doses.
2. Anticonvulsant action (especially on strychnine-induced seizures) and relieving action on spastic states.
3. Effectiveness following both oral and parenteral administration.
4. Rapid reversibility of effects.

When one considers the clinical results, a rather poor correlation exists between the effects of these drugs on the motor system and their anxiolytic properties. Indeed, it is quite clear that meprobamate is a better anxiolytic than other substances that cause muscular relaxation of equal intensity and duration in animals. For this reason, studies were carried out in an attempt to develop laboratory tests that could be more indicative of a tranquilizing effect in man.

Within this framework, consideration must be given to laboratory investigations in which the various myorelaxants were tested on experimentally-produced disturbed behavior in animals. The tests are of two types. The first studies animal interactions, and in particular their hostility and aggression; the second utilizes various conditioning procedures and especially those leading to states of fear and/or conflict.

An attenuation of natural viciousness (in monkeys) and of experimentally induced aggressiveness (in septal rats or isolated mice) has been described for meprobamate. This effect, however, is probably not specific; in fact, it appears only at doses that affect motor coordination and muscle tone. The methods of Pavlovian conditioning or conditioned avoidance have not been clearly useful in the identification of tranquilizing agents. These drugs, in fact, leave conditioned responses unaffected. The drugs are active, instead, when tested in various situations of conditioned suppression, in which a variety of aversive or painful stimuli are used to suppress ongoing behavior. If cats are given a shock whenever they attack a mouse, after a few trials they do not exhibit their normal aggression towards the mouse; meprobamate (20 mg/kg) restores this natural behavior, so that the animal will attack mice despite the electric shock. Similarly, meprobamate is effective in conflict behavior tests, such as that described by Jacobsen (1957). Cats are trained to open a food box; in some cases an air blast is associated with the opening of the box. This disrupts their behavioral pattern in opening the box; administration of meprobamate in these cats normalizes the feeding behavior. Several examples of this kind could be presented, and for more details on all these behavioral tests, the reader is referred to a review by Berger (1966). It should be noted, however, that these techniques, because of their complexity, hardly lend themselves to a preliminary assessment of new compounds; a screening test should be simple, so that many compounds can be evaluated.

The effect of the myorelaxant drugs on both spontaneous and evoked electrical brain activity has been extensively investigated. The present exposition will deal with the EEG effects of meprobamate, comparing them to the effects of other myorelaxants, in order to point out correlations, if any, between behavioral tranquilization and alterations in brain electrical activity.

A change to a higher-voltage, slower-frequency record was observed in the rabbit (Longo, 1962) with relatively high doses of meprobamate (50–100 mg/kg). In cats, a similar slowing of the waves was observed at the same dosage level (Gangloff, 1959; Funderburk and Unna, 1953). It is important to note that these changes are not similar to those observed during sleep. Studies on the effects of meprobamate on the electrocortical responses to reticular stimulation have demonstrated that this drug does not have a marked influence on the arousal reaction. With large doses, a particular modification of the morphology of the electrocortical arousal appears, which consists of a diminution in frequency and an increase in amplitude of the waves (Figure 3.6). Domino (1955) was the first to observe this reaction with mephenesin and gave the name *deactivation* to this pattern. It should be noted that this pattern is not characteristic of myorelaxant drugs, since it can also be seen following administration of subhypnotic doses of barbiturates.

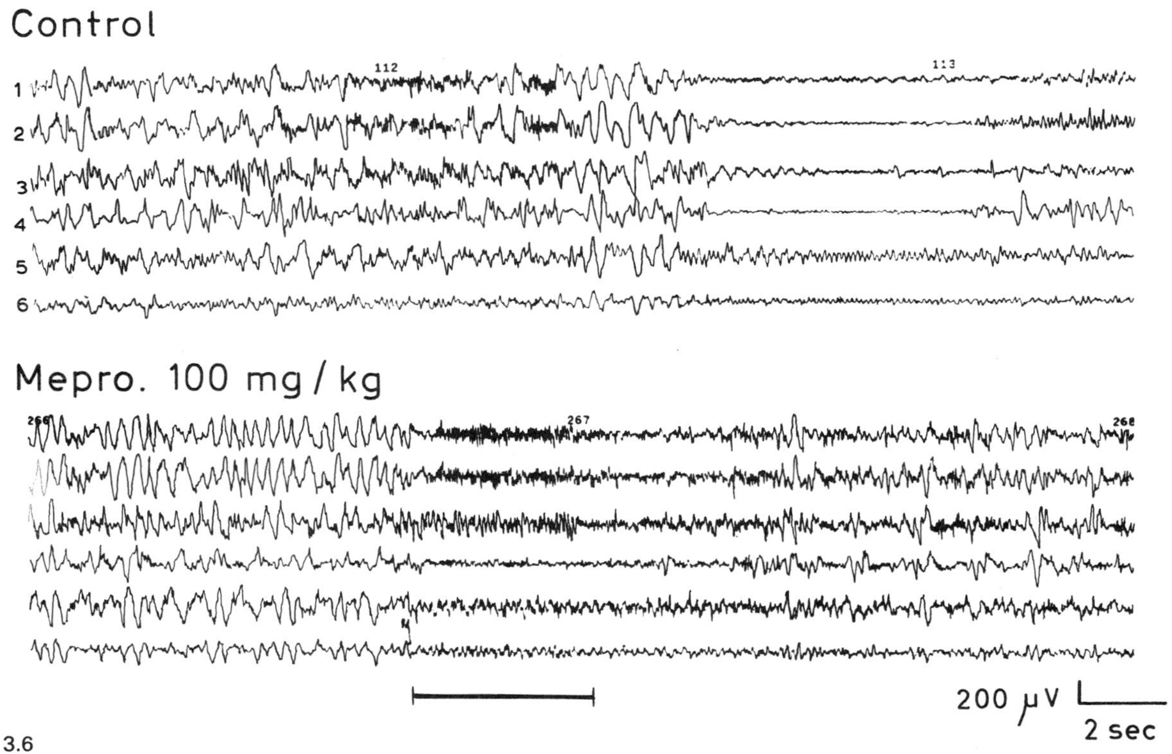

Figure 3.6

Effect of meprobamate on the cerebral electrical activity of the rabbit. The *upper tracing* shows the EEG at rest and after an acoustic stimulus (*bar*), which induces an activation. The *lower tracing* was registered 10 minutes after 100 mg/kg. i.v. Note the increase in slow waves; the acoustic stimulation now elicits a characteristic response (deactivation), which consists of waves with higher voltage and lower frequency than those in the control tracing.

Leads: (1) left anterior sensorimotor cortex; (2) right anterior sensorimotor cortex; (3) right posterior sensorimotor cortex; (4) right optic cortex; (5) anteromedial nuclei of the thalamus; (6) reticular mesencephalic substance (modified, from Longo, 1962).

Another effect brought out by the stimulation experiments is the inhibition of the recruiting response induced by the low-frequency stimulation of the anteromedial thalamic nuclei (Figure 3.7). This effect is observed with many myorelaxants (mephenesin, meprobamate, phenaglycodol) in doses that do not significantly modify the spontaneous tracing (King, 1956; Gangloff, 1959). Unlike the previously described effects, this one is not shared with the barbiturates, which often enhance the recruiting response (Domino, 1955; King, 1956).

The electrophysiological effect of these drugs is clarified by new concepts that have emerged from experiments dealing with the organization of the reticular activating system. In fact, the older, much-too-simple scheme of the activating role of this stystem has been modified by the demonstration (by means of stimulation and destruction experiments) of "deactivating" or "synchronizing" centers within this system (Figure 3.8). Low-frequency stimulation of the region of the *nucleus solitarius* in the medulla evokes a marked synchronization of the EEG; a small dose of thiopental in the vertebral artery, which supplies the blood to this region of the brainstem, produces an electrocortical arousal because the drug abolishes the tonic synchronizing influence of these centers; similarly, a continuous EEG arousal is present in the so-called midpontine pretrigeminal preparation of the cat, in which this tonic influence is stopped by the surgical section. All these data point to the existence of centers, localized in the lower brainstem, that are responsible for a tonic synchronizing influence on the cortical activity (Moruzzi, 1964). In evaluating the EEG effects of meprobamate and of the other myorelaxant drugs, we must consider the influence of these drugs on both the caudal and the rostral centers of the reticular formation. The myorelaxant effect may depend upon the influence of the drugs on the caudal center, which, when blocked, causes cortical desynchronization. Therefore, this could explain why some benzazole derivatives or diethylpropanediol, which also possess myorelaxant properties, cause activation of the EEG (Funderburk et al., 1953). Other substances such as meprobamate, mephenesin, and, above all, carisoprodol, have influence on the rostral reticular centers (reticulocortical and thalamocortical diffuse pathways), causing the appearance of low-frequency, high-voltage waves.

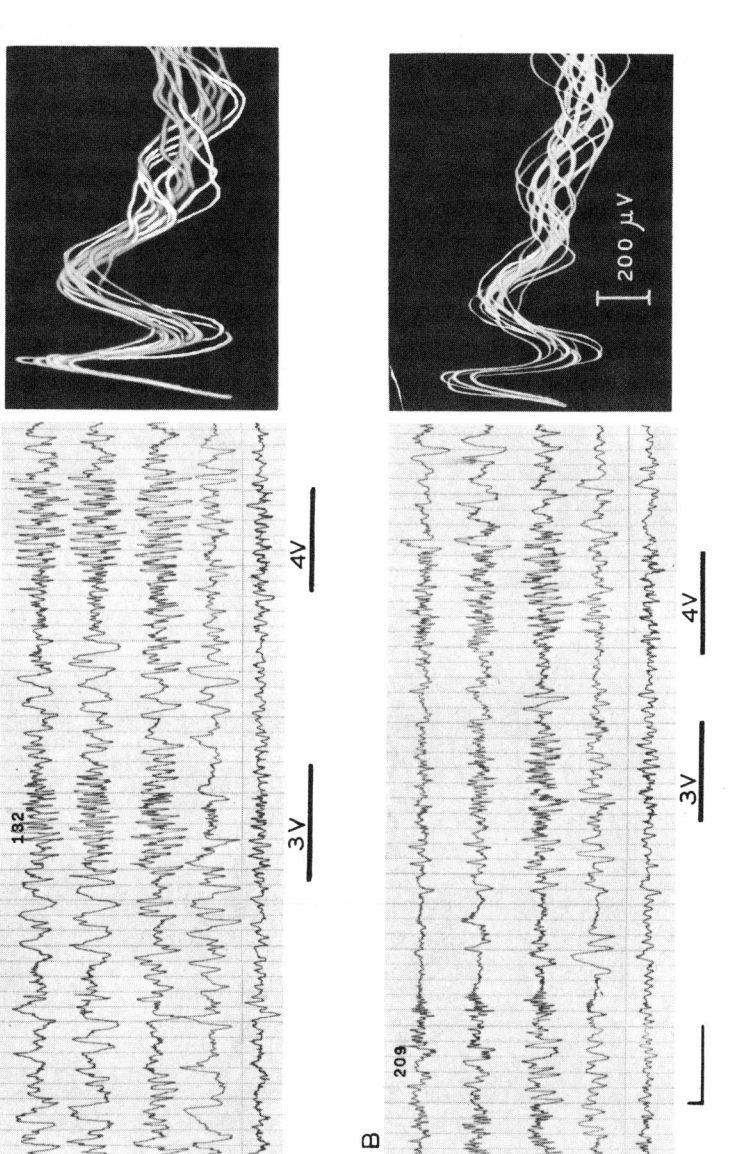

Figure 3.7

Effect of meprobamate on the recruiting response. **(A)** Recruiting induced by electrical stimulation (bars) of the thalamic anteromedial nucleus. **(B)** 10 min after 15 mg/kg of meprobamate, the response is inhibited. The tracings on the right are oscillographic recordings (sweep duration 150 msec) of the response to the 4 v stimulation, registered from the left anterior sensorimotor cortex. Square-waves stimulation of 1 msec duration, 6 c/sec. *Leads:* **(1)** R. anterior sensorimotor cortex; **(2)** L. anterior sensorimotor cortex; **(3)** L. posterior sensorimotor cortex; **(4)** L. optic cortex; **(5)** reticular mesencephalic substance. Calibration: 2 sec., 100 μv. (From Longo, 1962.)

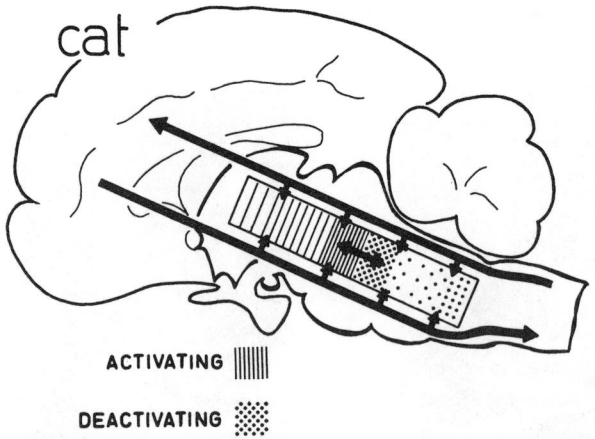

Figure 3.8
Activating and deactivating centers in the brainstem. Sagittal section
of the cat's brain, showing the reticular formation receiving afferents
from the periphery and from rostral centers. Besides the activating
system (*hatched areas*), there are deactivating (synchronizing)
structures (*stipled areas*), which are located caudally. In addition
to their influence on electrogenesis, these centers also play an
important role in modulating motor responses (from Rossi, 1965).

Other experiments have dealt with stimulation of the limbic
structures (hippocampus, septum, amygdala), which supposedly are
concerned with emotional behavior. Electrical stimulation of these
areas produces an afterdischarge of high-amplitude waves with a
frequency of 3–15 c/sec, which spreads throughout the limbic
system and is usually not accompanied by gross behavioral alterations. Meprobamate and tybamate shorten the duration of the
seizure, and carisoprodol does not affect it.

On the basis of the EEG findings, it is difficult to tie in any
relationship between the EEG pattern and the myorelaxing or tranquilizing activity. Some data, however, can be commented upon.

1. Analogies exist between the EEG pattern caused by some
myorelaxants (for instance, meprobamate) and that caused by
the barbiturates, i.e., the *deactivation* pattern, which probably
depends upon a combined effect upon the rostral and caudal
part of the reticular formation (see above).

2. The slowing of the cortical waves seen following administration of several myorelaxants (mephenesin, meprobamate, carisoprodol) is not similar to the EEG picture of sleep or drowsiness. This pattern, and the blockade of the EEG-arousal reaction caused by high doses of these drugs, are not in direct relationship to their tranquilizing properties. The most active in this respect is carisoprodol, which does not possess, in relation to the others, superior sedative activities. On the other hand, the slowing of the EEG could not be related to the myorelaxing properties, since drugs of this group, such as benzazole derivatives, induce activation of the EEG.

3. Inhibition of the electrical afterdischarge elicited by the stimulation of the limbic system is observed after administration of many of these drugs. This effect can be considered as a mild anticonvulsant action and is also shown by such compounds as barbiturates or diphenylhydantoin.

THE BENZODIAZEPINES

For almost five years meprobamate and similar drugs were the only available compounds for the treatment of the neuroses. Around 1960, clinical trials were begun with a new compound, developed in the American laboratories of the Roche Pharmaceutical Company. This compound, first given the nonproprietary name of methaminodiazepoxide and later changed to chlordiazepoxide, was eventually marketed under the trade name of Librium and belonged to a new chemical series, the 1-4-benzodiazepines, that up to that time did not have any clinical application. As can be seen from the formula (Figure 3.9), the benzodiazepine nucleus consists of a benzene ring and a seven-membered ring containing two nitrogen atoms in the positions 1 and 4; all the psychoactive derivatives of benzodiazepine also have a phenyl ring or pyridine ring as substituents.

The story connected with the development of this chemical series, as presented by Sternbach et al. (1964), is in retrospect very interesting. A group of compounds known as 3, 1, 4-benz*ox*adiazepines was selected for investigation mainly because of practical considerations. In this molecule, the seven-membered ring was supposed

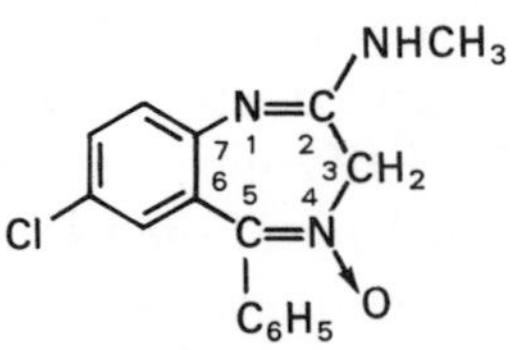

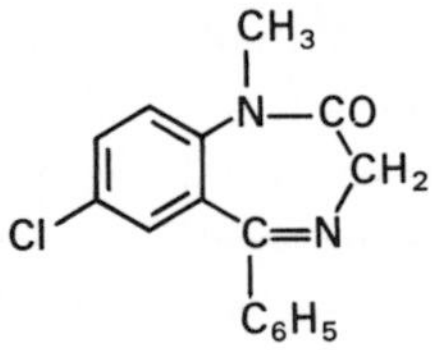

Chlordiazepoxide   Diazepam

Figure 3.9

to include an oxygen atom in the 3 position. Only a few members of this group were known, thus giving the chemist a wide field for exploration; moreover, the nucleus lent itself to the preparation of a large number of derivatives, with good yields. While the synthetic work was in progress, doubts arose about the identity of the compounds assumed to be benzoxadiazepines, and by a sequence of reactions, the true structure of the various compounds was finally established as 1-4-benzodiazepines, i.e., without the oxygen in the ring. The pharmacological screening demonstrated that several of these compounds possessed sedative, muscle-relaxing, and anticonvulsive properties, i.e., a spectrum of activity similar to that of the meprobamate group. However, chlordiazepoxide was consistently much more potent than meprobamate in various tests (Randall et al., 1960). On the basis of these results, chlordiazepoxide was tested in humans in various psychoneurotic states, with positive results. Shortly thereafter, another benzodiazepine was introduced into the clinic, diazepam (Valium), which proved to be more active than chlordiazepoxide. Since then, many other compounds of the same series have been marketed; presently, there are at least half a dozen of these available.

Clinical Effects

The therapeutic applications of the benzodiazepines are much the same as those for meprobamate: anxiety states, phobic reactions, alcoholism. The daily doses used in these states vary from 20 to 50 mg for chlordiazepoxide and from 10 to 30 mg for diazepam; these drugs are always given orally. Ten years after their clinical introduction, the benzodiazepines are acclaimed as superior to the drugs of the meprobamate group in the treatment of neurotic patients. Reliable and convincing data on this superiority are scarce; however, if the number of prescriptions filled in the drug stores reflects any efficacy of the compounds, it is unquestionable that at present the benzodiazepines are better than the other group.

In addition, their use has been extended to the treatment of epileptic patients, mainly as adjunctive therapy, and of sleep disturbances. The good results observed in epilepsy are not only due to the specific anticonvulsant effects, but also to the positive influence on the personality. The benzodiazepines were found to ameliorate slowness, perseveration, motor restlessness, and altered emotional response of these patients, and from a survey of the relevant literature one can conclude that the only factor against large-scale use in this field is the short-lasting anticonvulsant effect of these drugs. In another epileptic syndrome, *status epilepticus*, the benzodiazepines, and especially diazepam, proved very useful. *Status epilepticus* is one of the more severe complications of the various clinical forms of epilepsy and consists of consecutive convulsive attacks following each other at very short intervals, accompanied by a stuporous state, and, at times, hyperpyrexia. Unless vigorous therapy is initiated rapidly, death may ensue. Intravenous administration of 10–20 mg of diazepam controls within a few minutes the motor and EEG signs of *status epilepticus* (Figure 3.10). According to some authors (Gastaut et al., 1965), diazepam is the drug of choice for the treatment of these cases, being more safe and effective than the compounds used previously (phenobarbital, chloral hydrate, procaine, etc.). Another benzodiazepine, nitrazepam (Mogadon) has been introduced in the treatment of sleep disturbances. Favorable reports are found in the clinical literature and, at present, this drug is widely used as a hypnotic. Nitrazepam is effective at oral doses of 5–10 mg, which makes this drug one of the most active among hypnogenic substances.

The repeated administration of therapeutic doses of the various benzodiazepines results in a certain degree of tolerance, which, however, seems to concern more the sedative-hypnotic effect than the

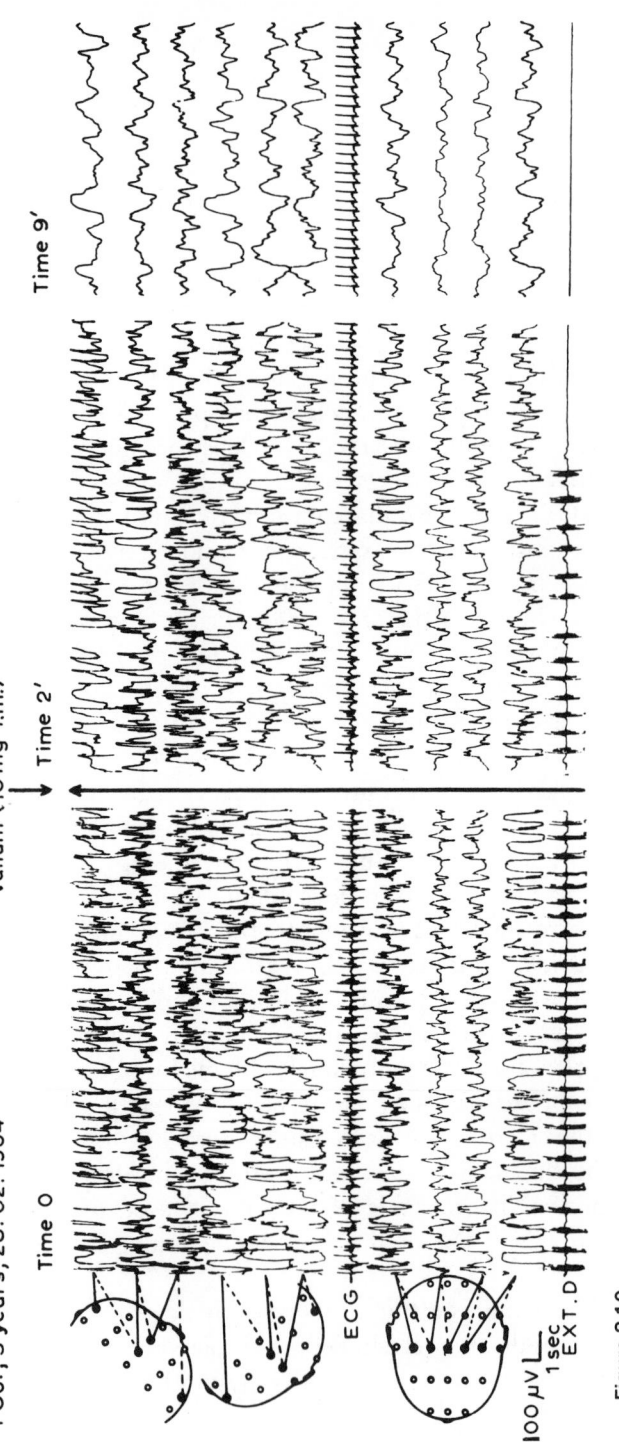

POU., 5 years, 28. 02. 1964

Valium (10 mg i.m.)

Time O   Time 2'   Time 9'

ECG

100 μV
1 sec
EXT. D

Figure 3.10

Severe *status epilepticus* in a 5-year-old child successfully treated with diazepam. The EEG shows continuous spike and wave complexes, accompanied by clonic motor convulsions. Two minutes after treatment the muscle clonic discharge (registered in **EXT. D**) stops; the electrical record is still abnormal. Nine minutes after, all the irritative elements disappear from the EEG, which shows only slow waves. The EEG leads are indicated in the scheme. **ECG**: electrocardiogram; **EXT. D**: electromiogram of the common extensor muscles of the right fingers. (From Gastaut et al., 1965.)

anti-anxiety effect. Also, the production of physical dependence has been described; the withdrawal signs were similar to those observed upon discontinuation of the sedative hypnotics or meprobamate.

Effects on Animals

The effect of benzodiazepines on gross behavior is very similar to that of mephenesin or meprobamate, therefore, it is not necessary at this point to describe it in detail (the reader is referred to the four points listed on page 81). However, it is worthwhile to discuss the differences between benzodiazepines and the other myorelaxants. The calming and taming effect on vicious or agitated animals is much more marked with benzodiazepines than with the meprobamate group. In the monkey, for instance, the scores for aggressive behavior are lowered at doses that have no influence on spontaneous activity or on muscle tone (Randall et al., 1961). A taming effect is also evident on septal rats: these rats with lesions in the septal region develop aggressive and vicious behavior; chlordiazepoxide is about ten times more potent than meprobamate in depressing the hyper-irritability of these animals (Schallek et al., 1962). These compounds also show a marked anticonvulsant activity. The antagonism to strychnine is particularly striking in diazepam. Although an antagonism against the chemical convulsants (pentamethylentetrazol, strychnine) has been described for all the myorelaxants, it appears only at high doses, and in most cases it only attenuates the convulsive manifestations and delays the death of the animal. In the case of diazepam, this antagonism is apparent at low doses (16 mg/kg, oral, in the mouse, according to Randall et al., 1961), which completely abolish the convulsions and prevent death. This anticonvulsant effect has been confirmed by various techniques (Bazinger, 1965) and has been described for other derivatives that have not yet been introduced in the clinic. Some have been found to be ten times more active than diazepam (Swinyard and Castellion, 1966).

The effect of the benzodiazepines on cerebral electrical activity has been studied mainly in cats and rabbits. From a survey of the data it seems that a certain difference exists between the two species.

In the cat, slowing of the EEG rhythms has seldom been observed (Randall et al., 1961; Schallek et al., 1964). More often, an increase in frequency of the waves has been reported (Réquin et al., 1963). In experiments in which behavior was observed, these EEG changes were accompanied either by restlessness and motor impairment (Schallek and Kuhen, 1965) or by a *relaxed wakefulness* (Hernandez-Péon et al., 1964); restlessness, ataxia, and EEG activation were also described for nitrazepam (Hernandez-Péon and Rojas, 1966; Schallek et al., 1964).

In the rabbit, slowing of the EEG waves has been often reported after administration of high doses of chlordiazepoxide, diazepam, and oxazepam (Monnier and Graber, 1962; Klupp and Kähling, 1965; Scotti and Longo, 1967). Cahn et al. (1964) in particular have described an increase of the spindle bursts and have suggested a relationship between the appearance of the spindles and muscular relaxation.

From the relevant experiments carried out in the rabbit and in the cat, it seems that the various benzodiazepines, at doses that cause slowing of the EEG rhythms, influence only slightly the EEG activation that follows either external stimulation or electrical stimulation of the reticular formation. Also in this case, however, there are reports (Gogolak and Pillat, 1965) that point to a rise in threshold after administration of nitrazepam (1–2 mg/kg) and diazepam (2–5 mg/kg) to the rabbit. In describing the action of nitrazepam on EEG arousal, these authors correlate it to the hynotic effect of the drug in man. (It should be noted in this regard that induction of sleep has not been described in animals treated with nitrazepam.)

The anticonvulsant effect of the benzodiazepines is well documented in EEG studies. Naquet et al. (1965) described an antagonistic action of diazepam towards the electrical and motor convulsive manifestations resulting from cicatricial lesions of the cat's cortex. Three benzodiazepines (chlordiazepoxide, diazepam, and oxazepam) were found to be effective in blocking the spikes and the Jacksonian convulsions caused by the topical application on the cortex of strychnine, nicotine, and morphine (Scotti and Longo, 1967).

Several investigations have been aimed at assessing the effect of these drugs on the electrocortical response obtained by stimulation of the amygdala and hippocampus, which are part of the limbic system and are concerned with emotional behavior. Electrical stimulation of these zones causes an EEG afterdischarge, usually restricted to the rhinencephalic structures and to the hypothalamus, but at times extending also to the cortex. All the benzodiazepines, to various extents, are active in inhibiting the afterdischarge. However, from a survey of the available data (Randall and Schallek, 1968), it is difficult to accept the effect of these drugs on the excitability of the limbic structures as a specific indicator of anxiolytic properties, since other anticonvulsants, such as phenobarbital or diphenylhydantoin show the same action. In this connection, it is interesting to note that a few years ago the latter drug had a short-lived use in the treatment of neurotic conditions; this use was probably due to similarities with the benzodiazepines found in some animal experiments (Cole and Davis, 1967).

CONCLUSION

Most of the agents described in this chapter have been reported to be clinically effective in reducing anxiety, tension, and other neurotic disturbances. Even so, there are many who continue to doubt whether these substances truly form a class of their own and who argue that "tranquilizers" were born only out of a contingent need to label the mild sedative effects noticed in the clinical trials at the beginning of the psychopharmacological era, when the attention of everyone was focused on finding specific treatments for every psychiatric disease. Considering in restrospect the fifteen years of history of the tranquilizers, one can conclude that these drugs do deserve a place of their own. If one analyzes the animal data, in order to draw some conclusions about their beneficial influence in emotional states, four basic effects can be set forth:

1. Relaxation of voluntary muscles.
2. Taming of spontaneous and elicited vicious behavior.
3. Beneficial effects on various types of conflict behavior.
4. Anticonvulsant action.

Within this frame of reference, a number of small differences can be detected among the various compounds, but the significance of these differences as related to clinical effectiveness cannot be stated. The clinical utility of these drugs probably is due to their combined effect on various central areas, so that a drug relieving muscle spasm, affecting the limbic system, and diminishing neuronal excitability is the best suited to interfere with the diversified symptoms that make up the neurotic syndrome.

References

Bazinger, R. F. *Arch. int. Pharmacodyn.* 154:131, 1965.

Berger, F. M. *Brit. J. Pharmacol.* 2:241, 1947.

Berger, F. M. *Pharmacol. Rev.* 1:243, 1949.

Berger, F. M. *J. Pharmacol.* 112:413, 1954.

Berger, F. M. In *Methods in Drug Evaluation,* ed. by P. Mantegazza and F. Piccinnini. North-Holland, Amsterdam, 1966. P. 218.

Berger, F. M., and Bradley, W. *Brit. J. Pharmacol.* 1:265, 1946.

Berger, F. M., and Schwartz, R. P. *J. Amer. Med. Assoc.* 137:772, 1948.

Cahn, J., et al. In *Neuropsychopharmacology,* ed. by P. B. Bradley, et al. Elsevier, Amsterdam, 1964. P. 490.

Cole, J. O., and Davis, J. M. *Psychopharmacology Bull.* 4:28, 1967.

Domino, E. F. *J. Pharmacol.* 115:449, 1955.

Domino, E. F. *Clin. Pharmacol.* 3:559, 1962.

Funderburk, W. H., and Unna, K. R. *J. Pharmacol.* 107:344, 1953.

Funderburk, W. H., et al. *J. Pharmacol.* 107:356, 1953.

Gangloff, H. *J. Pharmacol.* 126:30, 1959.

Gastaut, H., et al. *Epilepsia* 6:167, 1965.

Gellhorn, E. *Perspectives Biol. Med.* 8:488, 1965.

Gilbert, A., and Descomps, R. *Compt. Rend. Soc. Biol.* 69:145, 1910.

Gogolak, G., and Pillat, B. *Progr. Brain Res.* 18:229, 1965.

Goodman, L. S., et al. *Federation Proc.* 2:80, 1943.

Hernandez-Péon, R., and Rojas, R. J. A. *Int. J. Neuropharmacol.* 5:263, 1966.

Hernandez-Péon, R., et al. *Int. J. Neuropharmacol.* 3:405, 1964.

Jacobsen, E. In *Psychotropic Drugs*, ed. by S. Garattini and V. Ghetti. Elsevier, Amsterdam, 1957. P. 119.

Jacobson, E. *Progressive Relaxation.* The University of Chicago Press, Chicago, 1938.

Kaada, M. R. *J. Neurophysiol.* 13:89, 1950.

King, E. E. *J. Pharmacol.* 116:404, 1956.

King, E. E., and Unna, K. R. *J. Pharmacol.* 111:293, 1954.

Klupp, H., and Käling, J. *Arzneimittel-Forsch.* (Drug Res.) 15:359, 1965.

Longo, V. G. *Electroencephalographic Atlas for Pharmacological Research.* Elsevier, Amsterdam, 1962.

Monnier, M., and Graber, S. *Arch. int. Pharmacodyn.* 140:206, 1962.

Moruzzi, G. *EEG Clin. Neurophysiol.* 16:2, 1964.

Naquet, R., et al. *EEG Clin. Neurophysiol.* 18:427, 1965.

Randall, L. O., and Schallek, W. In *Psychopharmacology. A Review of Progress*, ed. by D. H. Efron. U.S. Dept. of Health, Education and Welfare, Washington, D.C., 1968. P. 153.

Randall, L. O., et al. *J. Pharmacol.* 129:163, 1960.

Randall, L. O., et al. *Current Therap. Res.* 3:405, 1961.

Réquin, S. et al. *Compt. Rend. Soc. Biol.* 157:2015, 1963.

Rossi, G. F. *Excerpta Medica, Int. Congr. Series* 93:117, 1965.

Schallek, W., and Kuhen, A. *Progr. Brain Res.* 18: 231, 1965.

Schallek, W., et al. *Ann. N.Y. Acad. Sci.* 96:303, 1962.

Schallek, W., et al. *Arch. int. Pharmacodyn.* 149:467, 1964.

Scotti, A., and Longo, V. G. *Arzneimittel-Forsch.* (Drug. Res. 17:1580, 1967.

Selling, L. S. *J. Amer. Med. Assoc.* 157:1594, 1955.

Sternbach, L. H., et al. In *Psychopharmacological Agents*, Vol. I, ed. by M. Gordon. Academic Press, New York, 1964. P. 137.

Swinyard, E. A., and Castellion, A. W. *J. Pharmacol.* 151:369, 1966.

CHAPTER 4

Hallucinogenic Drugs

Peyote high is something like benzedrine high. You can't sleep and your pupils are dilated. Everything looks like a peyote plant. I was driving in the car with the Whites and Cash and Pete. We were going out to Cash's place in the Lomas. Johnny said: "Look at the bank along the road. It looks like a peyote plant."

I turned around to look, and was thinking, "What a damn silly idea. People can talk themselves into anything." But it did look like a peyote plant. Everything I saw looked like a peyote plant.

W. BURROUGHS, *Junkie*

Man's use of substances that induce sublime or terrifying visions and fantasies dates back many thousands of years. It is of interest that man has not only looked to nature for substances to cure his bodily ills but that he also has searched diligently for drugs to relieve the disquietudes of his soul.

In the past, the so-called hallucinogenic drugs were employed in the religious and therapeutic practices of certain ethnic groups.

Extensive records describe the procedures and rituals governing their use.

In recent years, a less discriminating use of drugs to induce visions and fantasies has spread to and encompassed social and cultural aggregates within modern societies. An immense amount of commentary has been devoted to the medical, social, and religious aspects of this practice.

One of the most controversial problems related to this type of drug use is that of naming the agents in question, as the range of psychic effects presents special difficulties. The term "hallucinogen" is perhaps most widely accepted, as it denotes a phenomenon (hallucinations) that is readily understood by all. Another term, "psychotomimetic," refers to the alleged property of these agents of inducing transient psychotic states. The name "phantasticum," proposed by Lewin (1924) and subsequently taken up by Stoll (1947) as he described the actions of LSD, is less scientific; however, this may be the term that comes closest to describing the actual reaction of the subject to the administration of such agents. The most recent name is "psychedelic," by which Osmond (1957) meant to suggest that the drugs in question expand the spectrum of our sensory perception and are thus "mind expanding."

The widespread, uncontrolled use of hallucinogenic drugs is a phenomenon strictly related to the times in which we live. In fact, some of these very agents have been known and used for a long time without attracting much attention.

The identification and synthesis of mescaline, a hallucinogenic substance extracted from a Mexican cactus, dates back to the first years of the century. Numerous and authoritative studies led to a full description of its action on the sensorium and on the psyche, and to the proposal of its employment in experimental psychiatry, whether for therapeutic or diagnostic purposes (Klüver, 1928). Nevertheless, this drug was neglected for many years, except for its use in a limited number of self-experiments as, for instance, by the artists of Paris at the beginning of the century.

The interest in hallucinogenics received new impetus when a group of Swiss investigators in the Sandoz Laboratories (Stoll, 1947) found that the synthetic diethylamide derivative of D-lysergic acid, better known as LSD, proved very potent in inducing hallucinations and personality disturbances. In fact, even today this drug is the most potent of all known hallucinogenics, as it is sufficient to administer one-tenth of a milligram or less to man to produce a long-lasting hallucinatory experience. In these last years we have witnessed a continued extension of the use, both lay and professional, of the hallucinogens and of the search for similar agents, whether in the laboratory, where a long series of lysergic-acid derivatives were synthetized, or in the area of botanical and ethnographic research. Among the many drugs that thus became available, we can list psilocybin, extracted from Mexican mushrooms used in rituals, and the amide of lysergic acid, which was synthetized in the Sandoz Laboratories and subsequently recognized as the principal component of the extract of *ololiuqui*, the indigenous name of the seeds of a Convolvulacea (*Rivea corymbosa*) used in magic and divination.

Altogether, two facts are salient today. Not only are many hallucinogenic substances available but also their use has become diversified, extending from medical practice to areas entirely unrelated to medicine. The vicissitudes met by certain former psychologists at Harvard University, enthusiastic proponents of psychedelic enlightenment, are well known, and articles appear frequently in popular magazines to keep us informed of the widespread use of the hallucinogens in various social milieux. Even before scientific reports appear, these popular articles describe the results obtained with drugs due to the efforts of underground chemists who provide the clandestine market with new compounds. Moreover, sophisticated users of "kick" drugs and hallucinogens continually search for the ideal, most potent drug, capable of giving the pure psychedelic, liberating, and transcendental experience (the "final fix" of Burroughs and Ginsberg, 1963).

MESCALINE (PEYOTE)

The inhabitants of the Rio Grande region of Mexico refer by the name of "peyotl" or "peyote" (these are the orthographic versions which phonetically express best the sound of the indigenous name) to a cactus (Figure 4.1) known since ancient times, which grows on the rocky and arid plateaux of this zone. There are several botanical

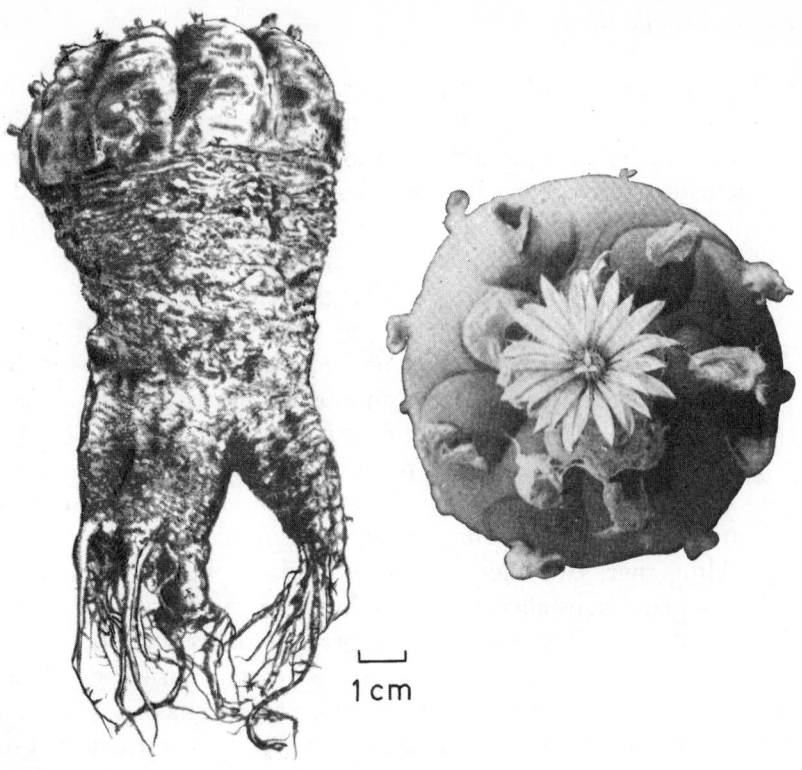

Figure 4.1
Photographs of the cactus peyote. The shape of this small plant resembles that of a molar tooth, since it exhibits a crown and a forked root (*left*). The light green crown is hemispherical, with several grooves. The figure at the right shows the cactus in bloom. Note the patches of whitish hairs; these hairs, particularly evident in the dry plant, suggested the name of the drug, in the local dialect, *peyote* means "white fuzz." (From Beccari, 1936; and J. Soulaire, *Cactus et Médecine*, Thiebaud, Paris, 1948.)

names for the plant, as it was named and renamed many times; generally the cactus is referred to as *Anhalonium williamsi* or *A. lewini*, as well as *Lophophora williamsi* or *L. lewini*.

The indigenous Indian tribes of Mexico (Mescaleros) and of adjacent parts of the United States used, and still use, the dried stem of the plant for their religious ceremonies. Local distributors of the drug call it "mescal buttons" and also, improperly, "mescal beans"; in the older literature the name "dry whiskey" was also employed. Rouhier (1927) reports that the price of the drug was 65 cents per kilogram in 1916. In 1936 Beccari states that the price was $3 per kilogram. Until a few years ago, some Texan horticulturists had peyote cactus available for the price of 8 cents apiece.

The initial research on the active components of the cactus was carried out at the end of the last century by German pharmacologists. On the occasion of Lewin's travels in the United States in 1887, he visited the Parke-Davis Laboratories, where he was given some mescal buttons, which he took back to Berlin. He undertook a pharmacotoxicological study of a crude extract of the buttons and he confirmed in the experimental animal its excitatory effect (Lewin, 1888). Investigations on the cactus were continued by Heffter, who proceeded systematically to find the active principles, extracting various chemical fractions (see Figure 4.2) and testing their effects in self-experiments. In 1897 he published a report, reaching the conclusion that mezcaline (or mescaline) is the substance responsible for the production of visual color hallucination; neither anhalonidine nor anhalonine or lophophorine had this effect. In subsequent studies, no less than eleven alkaloids were identified and studied pharmacologically: three that belong to the phenylethylamine group, among which was mescaline, and eight that were isoquinoline derivatives, among which was lophophorine (Reti 1953, 1954). Again these studies confirmed the fact that mescaline was the only one of the alkaloids that exhibited hallucinogenic properties.

Effects on Man

The Old World was made aware of the use of peyote at the time of the Spanish conquest, and the Spanish chroniclers provided the first account of its uses. For the primitive tribes of Mexico, peyote was a sacred plant, domicile of a god, and an object of veneration. The cactus constituted the most important element in their religious rituals, it could be harvested only at predetermined times of the year, and the harvest was surrounded by special ceremonies. Subsequently, it was consumed as a decoction or as an extract in the course of feasts or in sacred ceremonies, to which the inebriant properties of the cactus conferred a particular character. From the description of the effect of the concoction on the Indians, it appears that, jointly with a toxic syndrome (which included nausea, emesis, horripilation,

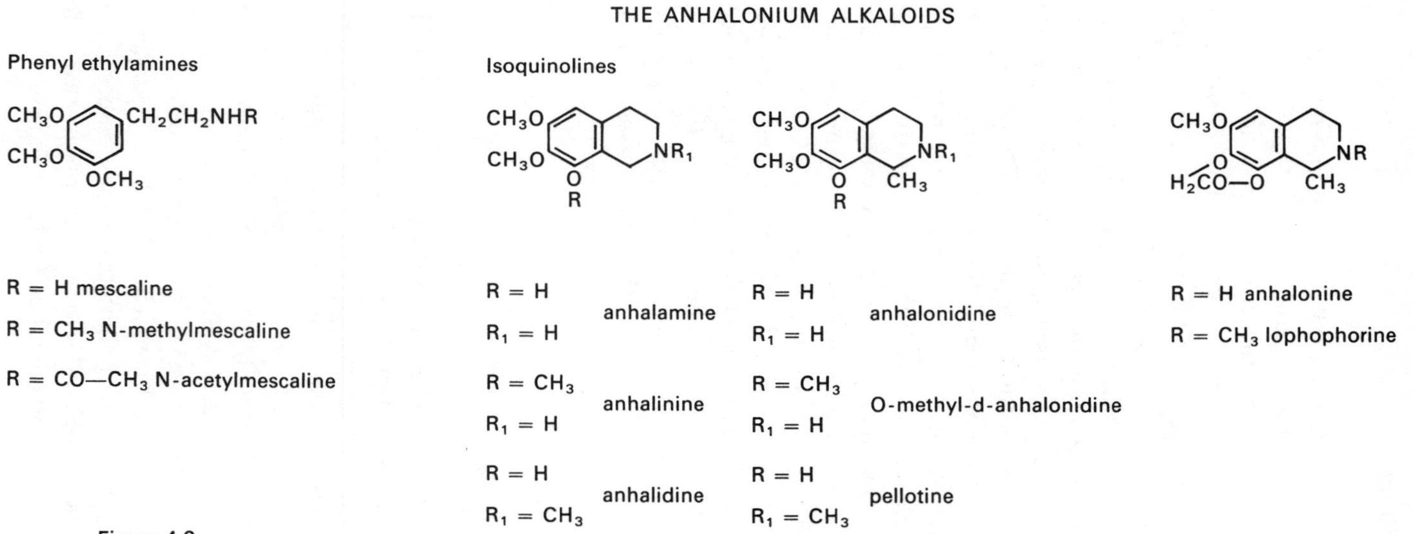
THE ANHALONIUM ALKALOIDS
Phenyl ethylamines
Isoquinolines
CH_3O
CH_2CH_2NHR
OCH_3
NR_1
NR
CH_3
$H_2CO—O$
R = H mescaline
R = CH_3 N-methylmescaline
R = CO—CH_3 N-acetylmescaline
R = H, R_1 = H anhalamine
R = CH_3, R_1 = H anhalinine
R = H, R_1 = CH_3 anhalidine
R = H, R_1 = H anhalonidine
R = CH_3, R_1 = H O-methyl-d-anhalonidine
R = H, R_1 = CH_3 pellotine
R = H anhalonine
R = CH_3 lophophorine

Figure 4.2
The alkaloids isolated from the cactus peyote (*Anhalonium williamsi*) can be classified into two chemical groups: three phenylethylamine derivatives, and eight isoquinoline derivatives. Mescaline is the only one which gives rise to hallucinations.

mydriasis) the major effect of the drug was on a psychic level, producing excitation, loss of the sense of hunger and thirst, and colorful visual hallucinations.

The use of peyote among the Indians has continued through many vicissitudes; the ritual was modified by the introduction of Christian symbolism. For example, the Indian tribes of Oklahoma founded in 1918 a Peyote Church, which united in a unique synthesis ancient Mexical rituals, Christian ceremonies, and finally, local customs. Today various Indian tribes continue to employ mescal buttons as a part of the rituals of the Native American Church which, according to a recent census, may include some 250,000 persons.

Since the studies of Heffter, it is known that mescaline is the compound responsible for the psychic effect of peyote. The administration, either oral or parenteral, of 0.2–0.5 g of this alkaloid suffices to induce the intoxication. Among the most characteristic symptoms is that of color hallucinations, generally agreeable in nature. Sensory illusions and transposition of sensorial excitation are also present: ordinary objects appear marvelous and strange, in beautiful and brilliant colors; sounds or noises are "seen" in color. In comparison, the impressions of everyday life seem pale and static. The psychic state can be better described as dysphoric than euphoric. Less frequent are hallucinations of other than the visual sensorium (auditory, proprioceptive). All these symptoms are accompanied—although to a lesser extent than following the ingestion of crude extracts of peyote—by side effects, particularly autonomic manifestations: bradycardia, nausea, headache, and sweating. These side effects are less evident when the drug is taken in divided doses.

It should not be thought, just because the hallucinogenic drugs became notorious recently, that mescaline was not a subject of early investigations. Copious literature exists both in the chemical and biological areas. As early as the paper by Heffter (1897) on peyote and mescaline, the hypothesis was advanced that the drug, especially because of its peculiar psychic effect, might become particularly tempting for *cultivirten Völkern*. Many neuropsychiatrists showed interest in the effects of this drug, and Klüver (1928) particularly compared the effects of mescaline on normal individuals with various psychotic syndromes. The conclusions of Klüver, which are shared by many students of the problem, were that the complex reactions obtained with the drug resembled schizophrenia much more than other pathological states. Among numerous subsequent investigations carried out on this problem, one of the most complete and authoritative is that by Osmond and Smythies (1952). In this context, it is interesting that the effect of mescaline on the schizophrenic proved to be more bland than that which the drug exerted on the normal subjects.

The various visual distortions and images experienced in the course of drug intoxication have been exhaustively described on the basis of interviews and illustrated by means of drawings and pictures. Generally, the descriptions, whether based on personal interviews or written by the subjects, are not considered adequate to fully describe the experience; even the drawings made by the subjects or those based on their descriptions scarcely suggest the subjective experience of the hallucinations; with this in mind, certain illustrations may be considered relevant. A drawing published by Marinesco (1933) constitutes a naive but faithful reproduction of a hand as it was seen during intoxication (Figure 4.3, *left*). This phenomenon seems to be characteristic; a more sophisticated drawing is shown at the right of Figure 4.3, illustrating alterations in body image during LSD intoxication. Délay et al. (1949) made an attempt to characterize, by means of a series of explanatory plates, the alterations of the spatial visual perception of colored objects, which these authors considered to be one of the most salient phenomena of the mescaline effect. Colors acquire a special intensity and meaning for the subject and they add an additional dimension to the subject's vision, causing objects and patterns to stand out in startling relief.

The possible effects of mescaline on artistic creativity aroused interest as soon as the effects of their drug on the sensorium became known. Studies carried out on professional painters had a twofold significance: on the one hand they yielded important information on possible drug influence on creative activity; on the other hand, they served as a more precise illustration of the hallucinatory visions that characterize the intoxication. This type of investigation was extended later to the other hallucinogens, such as LSD and psilocybin (Figure 4.3B). These results were both surprising and unequivocal. The artists were generally not satisfied with their own representation of their hallucinations, as they were drawn and painted under the drug influence. In fact, artists did not recognize, *post factum*, the

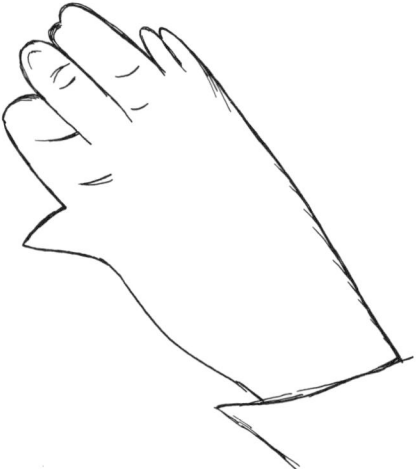

Figure 4.3
(A) Drawing of a hand made under the influence of mescaline, illustrating the phenomenon of megalo- and macropsia (Marinesco, 1933).

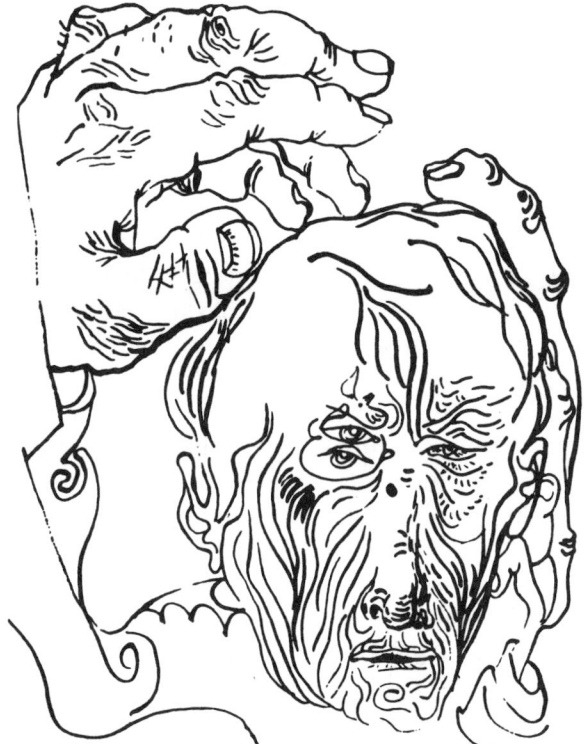

(B) The phenomenon of alteration in the appreciation of the body extremities is illustrated in a sophisticated way by a professional painter. This drawing was executed by a well-known Czech artist after the recovery from LSD intoxication (courtesy of *Panorama Sandoz*).

relationship between the experience and its pictorial result. Evident-
ly, the intoxicated subject stops hallucinating as he engages in artistic
activity, and he cannot paint or draw at the very moment he is
hallucinating. It might be concluded that the creative act and the
hallucinations cannot coexist and that they influence each other only
in the sense that the picture made can trigger off a new reverie or a
new hallucination. The artistic product with a delirious cachet,
which one might expect, cannot be realized in practice. All this not-
withstanding, the use of hallucinogens recently became popular in
artistic circles, and it gave rise to "psychedelic art"; yet it is far from
proven that this art is a true representation of the hallucinogenic
experience.

Effects on Animals

Mescaline is relatively nontoxic. Given intraperitoneally, its median
lethal dose in rats is 370 mg/kg. The symptoms of acute intoxication
may be divided into two phases: the earlier phase is characterized by
mild autonomic disturbances; the second phase includes the effects
upon the central nervous system, generally depressive in nature. In
the second phase, dogs and cats are rendered docile and tame (Sturtevant and Drill, 1956); catatonic behavior was described in rats,
accompanied by hyperreactivity to noises (Speck, 1957). In mice,
compulsive scratching has been described (Fellows and Cook,
1957). This syndrome is antagonized by chlorpromazine and morphine but not by the barbiturates. After high doses of mescaline, the
responses to painful stimuli are diminished, and depression and catatonia ensue (Sturtevant and Drill, 1956).

Early data, obtained in the prepsychopharmacology era by a
French investigator, pointed out a peculiar effect of the drug on the
behavior of conditioned animals. Rats were trained in a Warner cage
to give a conditioned-avoidance response to an auditory signal followed by an electric shock. Under the influence of the drug (100
mg/kg), they reacted to the sound as though it were the unconditioned stimulus: when the signal for the shock was given, they
howled as though they were being shocked (Sivadjian, 1934). This
accentuation of "emotional" vocalization to the conditioned stimuli,
was later confirmed in rats and in dogs (Bridger and Gantt, 1956)
trained to flex a leg to a tone. Under the effect of the drug (35 mg/

kg, subcutaneous) they responded with cries to both the conditioned and to the unconditioned stimulus (electric shock to the paw). Later works do not mention this phenomenon: Chorover (1961) for instance, studied the effect of mescaline (25 mg/kg) on the extinction period of a conditioned-avoidance response (in a shuttle box). The drug provoked an immediate and persistent suppression of the response.

Studies of mescaline on the cerebral electrical activity are relatively scarce. According to Speck (1958) low doses of mescaline (50 mg/kg) increases the low-voltage fast activity in the EEG of the rat; bursts of spikes appear at extremely high doses (200–400 mg/kg). Monnier and Krupp (1960) described a pattern of activation after 25 mg/kg. Baran and Longo (1965), using the same animal, described activation at low doses (25–75 mg/kg, intravenous) but the appearance of slow waves with higher dosages (up to 150 mg/kg). The latter authors emphasized the disappearance, after high doses, of the hippocampal theta rhythm; this phenomenon, observed also with other hallucinogens, will be commented upon later.

Compounds Related to Mescaline: Methoxyphenylethylamines and Methoxyphenylisopropylamines

Given the structure of mescaline, many analogs (see Figure 4.4) have been synthesized, and their properties have been investigated both in the laboratory and in the clinic. Smythies et al. (1967a) have studied mescaline analogs in rats, using two behavioral indices: the shuttle-box conditioned-avoidance response and the Sidman avoidance schedule. Mescaline, which is characterized by the 3-4-5 position of the methoxy groups (III) showed activity in these tests; the addition of one or two methoxy groups progressively increased the effect (V, VI). On the other hand, mescaline isomers, in which the position of the methoxy groups were changed (IV), showed no activity. Similarly, activity was decreased in the case of dimethoxy and monomethoxy compounds (I, II). It is interesting that there is an analogy between the results obtained employing the two experimental psychology tests and the psychotomimetic effect in man; for instance, Hollister and Friedhof (1966) have shown that the dimethoxy compound (II) was devoid of psychotomimetic activity in man.

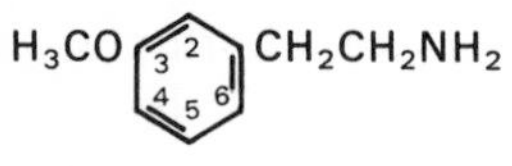

Figure 4.4
Structure-activity relationships of various methoxylated phenylethylamine analogs of mescaline have been studied both in laboratory animals and in man. The compounds **II** and **IV**, for instance, are devoid of hallucinogenic activity. (For further comments, see the text.)

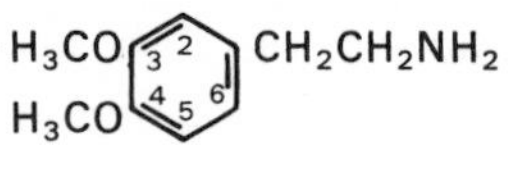

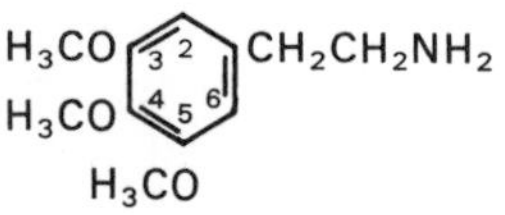

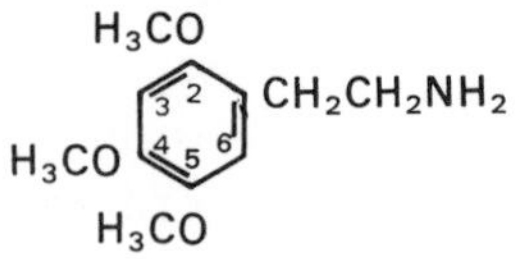

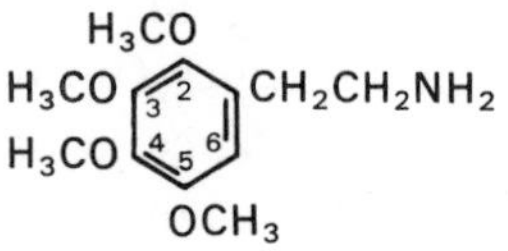

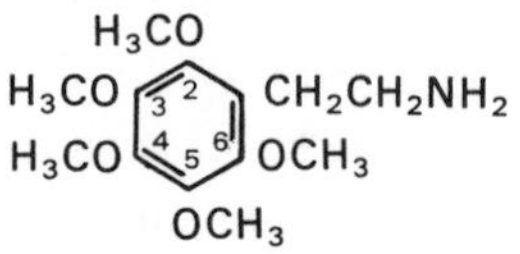

Another modification of the mescaline molecule is the introduction of a methyl radical in the alpha position of the side chain, which leads to compounds structurally related to amphetamine (Figure 4.5). The 3-4-5-trimethoxyamphetamine (TMA) produces in man a psychotomimetic response similar to that of mescaline, but with a stronger emotional component. Another analog, the 3-methoxy-4-5-methylendioxyamphetamine (MMDA) proved even more active than TMA. The lengthening of the aliphatic side chain of TMA and the enlargement of the heterocyclic ring of MMDA results in decreased psychotomimetic activity (Shulgin et al., 1961; Shulgin 1966). Other methoxy-substituted amphetamine analogs studied in rats by Smythies et al. (1967b). Unlike the mescaline derivatives, dimethoxy and methoxy substitutes did disrupt a conditioned response of the rat. As a matter of fact, the most active compound was *p*-methoxyamphetamine. According to these authors, substitu-

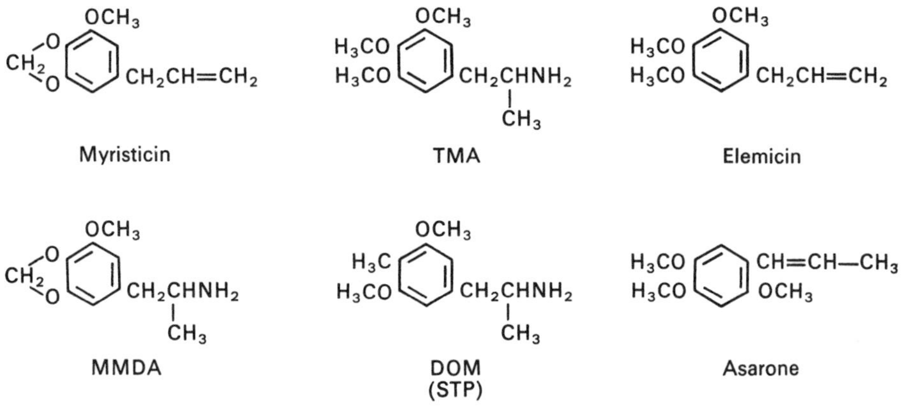

Figure 4.5
TMA, MMDA, and DOM are psychotomimetic in man. According to Shulgin (1966), the myristicin and elemicin present in nutmeg oil could be transformed in the body, respectively, into the active compounds MMDA and TMA. On the other hand, asarone, found in *Acorus calamus*, possesses only sedative properties.

tion in the para position of an amphetamine ring causes the appearance of "psychotomimetic" action in the rat. This compound also exhibits psychotomimetic activity in man (Shulgin et al, 1969).

STP, DOM

The hallucinogenic and psychodysleptic qualities of 2-5-methoxy-4-methylamphetamine or DOM (Figure 4.5) were probably discovered in the San Francisco "hippy" district by some sophisticated drug taker. Due to the state of excitement and elation it provokes, the drug was baptized with the name "STP," which is the trade name of a fuel additive (Scientifically Treated Petroleum) that is said to increase the pep and power of car engines. This substance was in use for quite a long time before it was chemically identified. Its effects were so well known and the unsuccessful attempts to antagonize overdosage disturbances with chlorpromazine was so widespread, that in areas of illicit drug use in large American cities, warnings were posted against using chlorpromazine as an antidote for the toxic effects of STP. Following studies of drug samples purchased on street corners by Government officials, STP was chemically identified and was the object of controlled human studies (Snyder et al., 1967). These studies demonstrated that the drug, ingested in doses of 10–15 mg, produces a reaction very similar to that of mescaline, but with more marked euphoric and excitatory components. Lower doses (2 mg) gave rise to an amphetamine-like syndrome. The duration of effect was 7–8 hours: thus the long-lasting reactions (up to three days) reported in the popular press were not confirmed. Also, the failure of chlorpromazine to antagonize STP was not substantiated by these authors, who found that chlorpromazine, in some instances, attenuated the effects of DOM. Pharmacological and toxicological studies of DOM are far from being complete. Its EEG and behavioral effect on rats, rabbits, and cats have been studied by Florio et al. (1969). Two phases of the action of the drug on the EEG and behavior could be differentiated in rabbits. Small doses (0.5 mg/kg) brought about a syndrome strongly resembling that induced by the sympathomimetic amines, with hyperpnea, mydriasis, startle reactions to external stimuli, horripilation, and lacrimal, salivary, and bronchial hypersecretions. Searching and exploration within the cage alternated with periods of stupor, during which the animal had a tendency to assume catatonic positions. This pattern was accompanied by cortical and subcortical activation with very evident theta waves at the hippocampal level. With higher doses (2–3 mg/kg), motor dysfunctions of the convulsive type appeared, first localized, with tremors of the limbs, blinking, grinding of the teeth, then involving the entire body. Tonic convulsions were never observed. The "grand mal" waves that repeatedly appeared in the EEG correspond sometimes to localized tremors and sometimes to clonic movements that never acquired severe intensity. Once the convulsive manifestations began, they continued for a long time, causing a state of deep prostration, which invariably led to death. Chlorpromazine, injected at the peak of the seizures, in doses varying from 2 to 5 mg/kg, intraperitoneally, did not prevent the progression of the intoxication or the death of the animal. On the other hand, the milder syndrome (of the sympathomimetic type) observed upon administration of the lower dosages (0.5 mg/kg) could be controlled by chlorpromazine. Upon intravenous administration of 2 mg/kg of this drug, the slow waves reappeared in the EEG, the animal calmed down, its pupils became miotic, and only the hyperpnea and the hypersecretion persisted.

The same toxic manifestations were seen in cats treated with 0.5 mg/kg, intraperitoneally; in addition, these animals showed evidence

Control

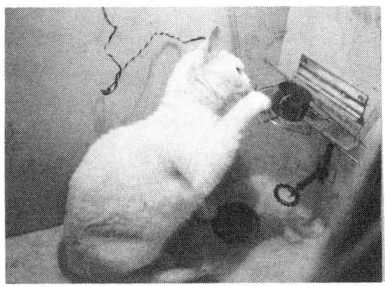

lever pressing

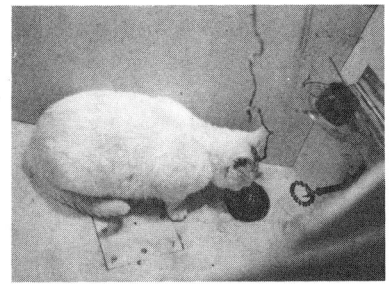

eating

DOM   0.5 mg/kg

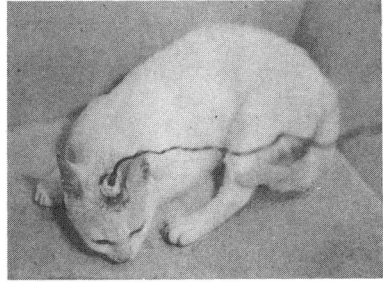

catatonic posture

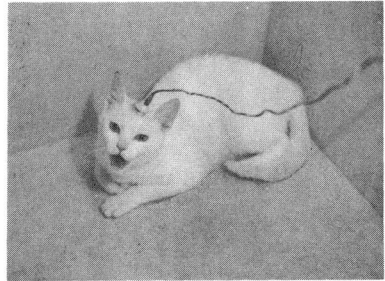

panting. mydriasis

Figure 4.6
Effects of DOM on animal behavior. The two upper photographs illustrate the behavior of a cat trained for an instrumental reward discrimination. Upon the presentation of a continuous sound, the animal presses the lever and eats. The two lower photographs illustrate some attitudes of the same animal treated with DOM; the performance of the response is disrupted, and the animal shows abnormal postures and stereotypes. The open mouth and protruding tongue, often observed in the course of the intoxication, resembles the attitude of a panting dog (from Florio et al., 1969).

of hallucinatory behavior: staring glaze, sudden jumps from one side to the other of the cage, and attempts to catch imaginary objects (Figure 4.6). The EEG studies revealed a rapid activity in the cortical leads, similar to the activation pattern, but of higher voltage. In the same animal, DOM (0.25 mg/kg) also proved able to disrupt conditioned discrimination.

Even though the clinical and animal results cannot be compared directly, one particular aspect of the results in animals is relevant to the results reported in man, that is, the alleged danger of using chlorpromazine to counteract an overdose of DOM. This danger was not confirmed by Snyder et al. (1967) who found, instead, that chlorpromazine was effective in attenuating the symptoms of DOM intoxication. However, the results obtained with animals suggest that chlorpromazine will not antagonize the toxic effects of DOM when this drug is administered in dosages large enough to elicit convulsions. The reasons for the inconsistency between the results of Snyder et al. (1967) and the previous warnings that went out to the black market clientèle may be that (1) only moderate dosages were given in Snyder's controlled human trials, and (2) the amount of DOM taken by drug users exceeds the dose that can be counteracted by chlorpromazine. It is also possible that STP pills contain some other ingredients that potentiate and prolong the intrinsic effect of DOM.

MYRISTICIN AND ASARONE

Myristicin is the main constituent of the oil extracted from nutmeg. This spice, freely available in grocery stores, is the dried kernel of the plant *Myristica fragrans*, native to the Molucca Islands. It is used, *faute de mieux*, by drug addicts and others seeking excitement and new experiences. Unpleasant side effects (vomiting, nausea, tremors, intense vasodilatation) are predominant in the intoxication, during which the subject may also experience euphoria, feelings of unreality, and changes in perception.

The few investigations carried out with myristicin in animals did not show any symptoms suggesting psychotomimetic or excitant effects. Careful chemical analysis of the oil extracted from nutmeg has shown, in addition to myristicin, the presence of another substance, elemicin, which may also be responsible for the central effects of the drug (Shulgin, 1966). An interesting hypothesis put forward by Shulgin is the transformation of these two compounds in the body into, respectively, trimethoxyamphetamine (TMA) and methoxymethylendioxyamphetamine (MMDA), which probably are responsible for the psychotomimetic syndrome (Figure 4.5).

The root of *Acorus calamus,* a plant that grows in Asia, Europe, and North America, is used in folk medicine as a euphoriant and bronchodilator. The active principle, asarone (1, 2, 4-trimethoxy-5-propenylbenzene) and β-asarone, were studied extensively in the laboratory (Das et al., 1962), but only tranquilizing properties were demonstrated, in addition to a potent spasmolytic effect. Asarone was found very active in antagonizing the stimulant effects of amphetamine and mescaline. This is of interest in view of the chemical similarities between asarone and amphetamine.

DIETHYLAMIDE OF D-LYSERGIC ACID (LSD)

In 1943, Albert Hofmann, a chemist at the Sandoz Laboratories in Basel, discovered the peculiar psychic effects of D-lysergic acid diethylamide (LSD). LSD is a semisynthetic, obtained in the laboratory by combining a natural product, lysergic acid, present in the extract of the fungus *Claviceps purpurea,* with diethylamide. Hofmann, after having accidentally ingested a fraction of one mg of LSD, experienced marked disturbances in perceptions, vivid visions of colored patterns, altered thinking processes, dizziness, and nausea. With further self-experiments, Hofmann confirmed the powerful hallucinogenic properties of the drug, and, thereafter, the pharmacologists at Sandoz reinvestigated the properties of LSD in animals. In fact, prior to Hofmann's dramatic finding, this drug, as well as other semisynthetic derivatives of lysergic acid, had been screened in the laboratory. LSD proved actually pharmacologically not very different from the parent compounds, for example, ergometrine (lysergic acid isopropanolamide). The only difference was that LSD showed a marked central effect, as exemplified by its exquisite effect on body temperature and its generalized excitatory action.

It should be stressed at this point that the psychic effect of LSD was discovered at the peak of wartime research, and the implications of the possible use of this potent drug in chemical warfare immediately became apparent. Accordingly, the first results were strictly classified, and only in 1947 did a clinical and pharmacological report appear in the literature (Stoll, 1947), describing the discovery of a novel "phantasticum"—a term employed by Lewin to describe the effects of mescaline. The main difference between LSD and mescaline was the extreme potency of the new compound, potency not yet excelled, although other substances with analogous effects have been discovered.

Effects on Man

Further research in man, carried out both in Europe and the United States outlined more clearly its psychological effects, defined the active dose, and compared its action on normal and psychotic individuals. A comprehensive listing of the relevant literature can be found in the book *The Hallucinogens* by Hoffer and Osmond (1967). The effective dose of LSD was evaluated as between 50 and 100 μg (about 1 μg/kg of body weight). Except for a more rapid appearance of symptoms upon parenteral administration, the effects of the drug are independent of the route of administration.

As in the case of mescaline, the symptoms of LSD intoxication can be subdivided in two categories. One series of effects is related to the autonomic nervous systems, and consisted of chills, sweating, mydriasis, nausea, headache, and dry mouth. Other effects are central in origin. Mood alteration is evident in the drugged person; reactions vary from euphoria to anxiety and depression, and are undoubtedly influenced by the person's personality and expectations.

The principal subjective symptoms are perceptual changes, in particular, visual distortions. Objects are perceived in the strangest ways, with clear-cut shapes and brilliant colors. Proprioceptive perception is also affected. If the subject looks at his own hand and lets his mind idle, a slow but continuous change of visual perceptions occurs; the outline of his hand becomes indistinct and its apparent form becomes altered. These distortions may be obliterated at any moment by the slightest effort to concentrate on his hand. Images and visions, appearing mainly when the eyes are closed, are always reported. These images are of an extraordinary complexity and plasticity, a kind of kaleidoscopic game of colors and shapes: fretwork, filigree, weird patterns like Christmas wrapping papers, spirals and dots always in movement. Because of this phenomenon, the drug has received the name *hallucinogenic*, even though the appearance of real hallucinations, i.e, formed images independent of external stimuli, are not common at usual dosages.

Auditory hallucinations are present in the form of musical chords, unusual sounds, and noises.

Intellectual processes are impaired, there is a certain difficulty in concentration and reasoning. Consciousness is not lost; the individual is aware of his state and, what is more remarkable, he can control his images and visions. Indeed, this peculiarity of LSD intoxication is usually not sufficiently stressed. The "hallucinogenic experience" clearly depends on the subject and on whether or not he wants to let himself go under the influence of the drug. This explains the variety of descriptions of the drug's effects, beginning with that of Rothlin, a Sandoz pharmacologist, when he stated that he never experienced hallucinations, but only a state of drunkenness and dysphoria (De Bold and Leaf, 1967).

The intoxication usually lasts from 6–8 hours and is followed by insomnia. Generally, the subject is completely recovered by the next day, except, naturally, for his memories of the pleasant or unpleasant episode. Therefore, a person who has had a pleasant experience will be more inclined to retake the drug than a person who has had an unpleasant experience. However, real dependence on the drug has never been described. It should be added here that there is a very rapid development of tolerance to LSD, so that an identical dose, taken two days in succession, will not cause the same effects. This tolerance is of a brief duration, and it suffices to let a few days pass for sensitivity to the drug to return.

LSD, like mescaline, produces milder effects in schizophrenics than in normal subjects. This was noted first by Stoll and later confirmed in several investigations. There is no proof, however, that a biological tolerance related to biochemical factors underlies the phenomenon; some authors attribute these milder effects to negativism, autism, and other psychological factors (Balestrieri, 1961).

Following the paths set thirty years earlier by the neuropsychiatric research with mescaline, researchers attempted to produce a temporary "model psychosis" with LSD. Indeed, in the case of LSD, just as in that of mescaline intoxication, certain traits were found that matched those of schizophrenia. Accordingly, one of the aims of the investigations was to determine, with LSD as a tool, the etiology of schizophrenia; simultaneously, LSD intoxication was employed as a method for finding new therapeutic agents for the treatment of this disease. In the course of these investigations, it was noticed that some individuals were able, under the influence of the drug, to verbalize the repressed components of their conflicts (abreaction). This finding suggested that LSD might be helpful in psychotherapy, and further research confirmed the value of LSD in facilitating access to withdrawn patients, in inducing episodes of catharsis, and in activating association and recall. These effects of LSD proved of value when the drug was subsequently used in the treatment of chronic alcoholism.

This discussion has so far centered on psychiatric applications of LSD, yet the majority of those who take LSD use it for quite different purposes. Man has always searched for new experiences and sensations. The particular aspect of LSD intoxication that is related to this search for novelty has been termed "psychedelic" by Osmond (1957); this term signifies the opening of the gates of the "psyche" to novel, previously unexperienced sensations. What has caused the spread of this particular drug, basically not distinct in its action from the actions of other drugs or procedures employed for millennia to obtain a similar "psychedelic" experience?

In an astute analysis of the motives that move a particular individual to seek ecstasy through LSD, Barron (1967) probably quite rightly attributed a special role to the enormous publicity in the popular press. There was no newspaper or magazine in Europe, in the United States, or in other parts of the world that did not help arouse interest in LSD by emphasizing the novel experiences produced by the drug.

Another factor that should not be underestimated is our present historical context: younger elements of society, in particular, favor the use of drugs that promise escape from their frustration and malaise. All those who have taken this drug and/or have had research experience with it agree that it has a unique effect—an effect that is independent of the identity of the taker. Statements such as "unforgettable," "indescribable," and "sublime" are frequently found in reports, and it can be easily understood why such testimonies should tempt individuals of the most divergent backgrounds to try LSD.

It should be stressed that, in spite of widespread use of the drug, chronic use or addiction to LSD is rare if it exists at all. Indeed, as varied as LSD experiences may be from person to person, the drug does not exhibit any of the analgesic and euphoriant properties that may cause the development of habituation. The overwhelming majority of those using LSD illicitly do so only a few times. Although there are no reports of fatalities due to the direct toxic action of the drug, the intrinsic features of LSD intoxication can have dangerous consequences. A state of acute paranoia and confusion may develop in some individuals, leading to aggressive behavior or suicide. Sometimes, the patient's reaction to the drug is prolonged, consisting of a kind of chronic anxiety that persists for weeks. Even though such effects have been described in borderline psychotics, the toxic potential of LSD is not insignificant and should be fully evaluated. Indiscriminate and unsupervised intake clearly presents hazards (Cohen, 1966).

The Psychotomimetic Activity of Other Lysergic Derivatives

Many derivatives of lysergic acid have been synthetized and examined in the laboratory and in the clinic in a search for correlations between (*a*) the structure of the LSD molecule and (*b*) the psychotomimetic effects. The results obtained by the group of clinical investigators at Lexington (Isbell et al., 1959) are presented in Table 4.1. Psychotomimetic activity is absent in the LSD isomers; similarly, the brom-substituted LSD is devoid of activity. Variations in the amide group or ring substitution with other radicals result in a diminution in psychotomimetic potency (Figure 4.7). It should be stressed that all the compounds of this series retain their potential for psychotomimetic activity. For instance, the butanolamide derivative of 1-methyl lysergic acid, which was carefully screened and then introduced into therapy for the treatment of migraine headaches and rheumatic pain, proved in some instances to produce hallucinations when used in very high dosages. On the other hand, the nonsubstituted amide of lysergic acid, found in the ololiuqui seed (see page 141), has calming properties (Solms, 1956).

Table 4.1 *Psychotomimetic and Antiserotonin Potencies of a Series of Lysergic Acid Derivatives*

Reference Number Shown in Figure 4.7 and Code Name	Compound	Dose Approximately Equivalent to 1.0 µg/kg of LSD-25	Relative Psychotomimetic Activity (LSD-25 = 100)	Relative Antiserotonin Activity (LSD-25 = 100)	Remarks
		A. *Stereoisomers*			
(1) LSD-25	d-Lysergic acid diethylamide	1.0	100	100	
(6) L-LSD	L-Lysergic acid diethylamide	>70	0	0	No psychotomimetic effect in doses used
(7) l-LSD	d-Iso-lysergic acid diethylamide	>50	0	0	No psychotomimetic effect in doses used
		B. *Variations in amide group*			
(2) DAM-57	d-Lysergic acid dimethylamide	10	10	23	Effect similar to LSD; onset quicker and course shorter
(5) LAE-32	d-Lysergic acid monoethylamide	20	5	12	Effect similar to LSD; course shorter
(3) LPD-824	d-Lysergic acid pyrrolidide	10	10	5	Effect similar to LSD; course shorter
(4) LSM-775	d-Lysergic acid morpholide	9	11	2	Effect similar to LSD; course shorter

C. Substitutions in ring system

(13) MLD-41	d-1-Methyl lysergic acid diethylamide	3	33	370	Effect similar to LSD; onset slower
(14) ALD-52	d-1-Acetyl lysergic acid diethylamide	1	100	210	Effect similar to LSD; course similar
(10) BOL-148	d-2-Brom-lysergic acid diethylamide	>86	<2	103	Only partial LSD effect; course shorter
(11) MBL-61	d-1-Methyl-2-brom-lysergic acid diethylamide	>175	<1	533	No psychotomimetic effect in doses used

D. Substitutions in rings and variations in amide

(16) MLA-74	d-1-Methyl-lysergic acid monoethylamide	25	4	835	LSD-like; short course
(17) ALA-10	d-1-Acetyl-lysergic acid monoethylamide	15	7	39	LSD-like; short course
(18) MPD-75	d-1-Methyl-lysergic acid pyrrolidide	>20	<5	130	Only partial LSD effect; short course

SOURCE: Modified, from Isbell et al., 1959

NOTE: See Figure 4.7 for structural formula.

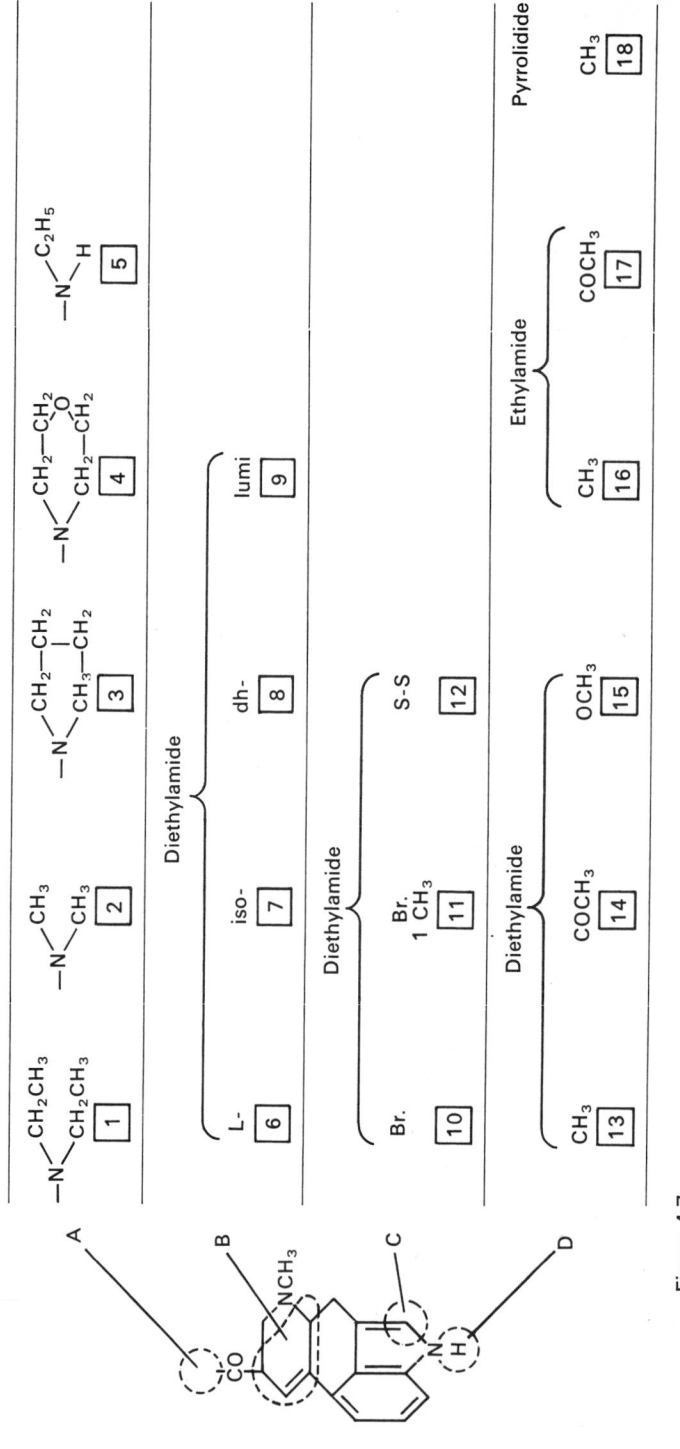

Figure 4.7

Chemical structures of some lysergic-acid derivatives. See Table 4.1 for their relationships with psychotomimetic activity. None of the variations in the amide group, shown in **A**, abolish the psychotomimetic effect, although they do affect its potency. Changes in the steric configuration or loss of the double bond, as exemplified in line **B**, lead to the disappearance on the specific effects in man. Inactive also are the compounds in which the hydrogen in **C** is substituted. On the other hand, chemical substitutions on the indole nitrogen (line **D**) give rise to compounds with psychotogenic effect. (From Cerletti, 1959.)

Effects of LSD on Animals

The terms "hallucinogen" and "psychotomimetic agent" are based on the behavioral and psychic effects of LSD in man; in the animal, the drug does not present any array of pharmacological effects that can be considered to be a counterpart of its action in man.

LSD was already on the chemical shelf at Sandoz prior to Hofmann's accidental intoxication, and it had already been tested on animals routinely. In the files, it was classified, together with other amides of lysergic acid, as a relatively weak uterine stimulant, a vasoconstrictor, and a central excitant.

Following Hofmann's discovery, new studies of this product were initiated; the results obtained cannot be considered satisfactory with regard to the ultimate explanation of the mechanism of its action in man. Regarding its basic mechanism of action, two major theories have been suggested. The first stresses the sympathergic effect of this molecule. Chemically, this drug has the structure of a sympathomimetic substance (because of the presence in the molecule of the phenylethylamine and of the tetrahydronaphtylamine skeleton) but also can be considered a sympatholytic compound of the ergotamine series.

The signs of acute intoxication have many points in common with the central sympathomimetic syndrome. In some animals, such as the rabbit, motor excitation and hyperthermia prevail; this is the E-syndrome (E=excitatory) of Cerletti (1959). However, in other animals, such as the dog and the cat, depression and, sometimes, a catatonic state occur. Autonomic disturbances also occur, especially after high doses: they consist of salivation, piloerection, mydriasis, hypertension, and vomiting. Certain actions differentiate LSD from other central stimulants. Among these are: hyperthermia, which is evident at doses comparable to those inducing hallucinations in man; hyperglycemia; inhibition of the genetic incoordination that is characteristic of a certain strain of mice (waltzing mice); and the augmentation of spinal reflexes.

LSD proved to be among the most toxic of all the synthetic and natural derivatives of lysergic acid. The lethal dose for rabbits is 0.3 mg/kg (intravenous), making the rabbit the most sensitive laboratory animal, but not the most sensitive animal of all, for 0.1 mg/kg sufficed to kill an elephant at the Oklahoma City zoo (West et al., 1962). LSD is also active in lower vertebrates, insects, and molluscs. The Siamese fighting fish (*Betta splendens*) placed in water containing 0.2 mg/l loses its aggressiveness; spiders spin their webs in disorganized patterns; the mystery snail shows deep motor alterations in water containing 0.01 mg/l. These effects, however, in themselves, can hardly be considered a criterion of hallucinogenic activity in man (Jacobsen, 1963).

The second theory, which stimulated a great deal of interest, attempted to tie the specific hallucinogenic properties of LSD to its antagonistic effect towards serotonin ($5HT$). Gaddum (1957) demonstrated a marked antagonism by LSD towards serotonin in isolated rat intestine, and he hypothesised that at the central level this antagonism constitutes the basis of the hallucinogenic action of LSD. The role of serotonin in the higher centers was proposed by Brodie (Shore et al, 1955) after large quantities of this amine were found in various brain areas. Additional pharmacological observations on the central effect of reserpine (which depletes the central stores of $5HT$) and of monoamineoxidase inhibitors (which prevent $5HT$ destruction) served to strengthen this view. The same concept of a role of $5HT$ in central integration was taken up and elaborated by Woolley (1962) to include a possible mechanism of the genesis of schizophrenia. Further research along this line has considered the antiserotonin effects of a series of LSD-related drugs, comparing them with their hallucinogenic properties. These results demonstrated that the antiserotonin action does not in itself constitute a reliable indicator of the hallucinogenic property: some substances, such as brom-lysergic acid diethylamide (BOL) or 1-methyl-lysergic acid butanolamide (UML), which manifest strong antiserotonin activity, have a slight, inconsistent psychotomimetic effect (see above, the clinical results of Isbell et al., 1969). Although it is a serotonin antagonist, LSD is, at slightly higher doses, a smooth muscle stimulant; moreover, many of its central effects are similar to those observed after administration of drugs that cause increased concentrations of serotonin to appear in the central nervous system (Mantegazzini, 1966). Recent contributions to this theory (Andén et al., 1968) brought evidence that BOL and UML are unable to mimic this serotonin-like central effect. Therefore, it should be taken into consideration that the central effect of LSD may just as well be due to its serotonin-like activity as to its antagonistic effect towards serotonin.

The problem of the central action of LSD has been approached also by means of neuropharmacological and neurophysiological techniques. The prominent sensory disturbances produced by LSD in man served as a point of departure for studies on the effects of the drug upon the electrical activities evoked at various sites of the afferent sensory pathways. Some of the described alterations, like the behavioral blindness of monkeys and cats, and the spontaneous action potentials in the electroretinogram, have been obtained with doses hundreds of times higher than those effective in man; the time course of the events was also not comparable. These results, obtained in anesthetized animals—whose sensory input was therefore obtunded— must be considered with some caution (see, for references, Jacobsen, 1963). The results obtained in unanesthetized animals are more acceptable. According to Key (1965), the responses evoked in the auditory pathways of cats with chronically indwelling electrodes show a spontaneous variability in amplitude and duration, related not only to the level of arousal but also to ambient sensory stimulation. Administration of small amounts of LSD (10 μg/kg) produces an increase in the variability of the responses. This phenomenon could be attributed to the influence of the drug on the neuronal organization that regulates the flow of afferent and efferent activities of the brain rather than on the pathways of specific stimulus conduction.

LSD also produces electroencephalographic changes in various laboratory animals. The rabbit, for instance, exhibits upon the administration of 20–50 μg/kg, a flattening of the corticogram and an almost complete disruption of the theta rhythm of the hippocampus (Figure 4.8); these changes are less evident in the cat; in this animal, the effect of LSD is limited to an activation of the tracing. Purpura (1956) has demonstrated an obliteration of the cortical response to repetitive electrical stimulation of the anteromedial thalamic nuclei (recruitment block); the "secondary" component of the sensory evoked potential was also blocked. This block could have been due, according to Purpura, to the effect of the drug on the cortical axodendritic synapses. However, as later demonstrated by Roth

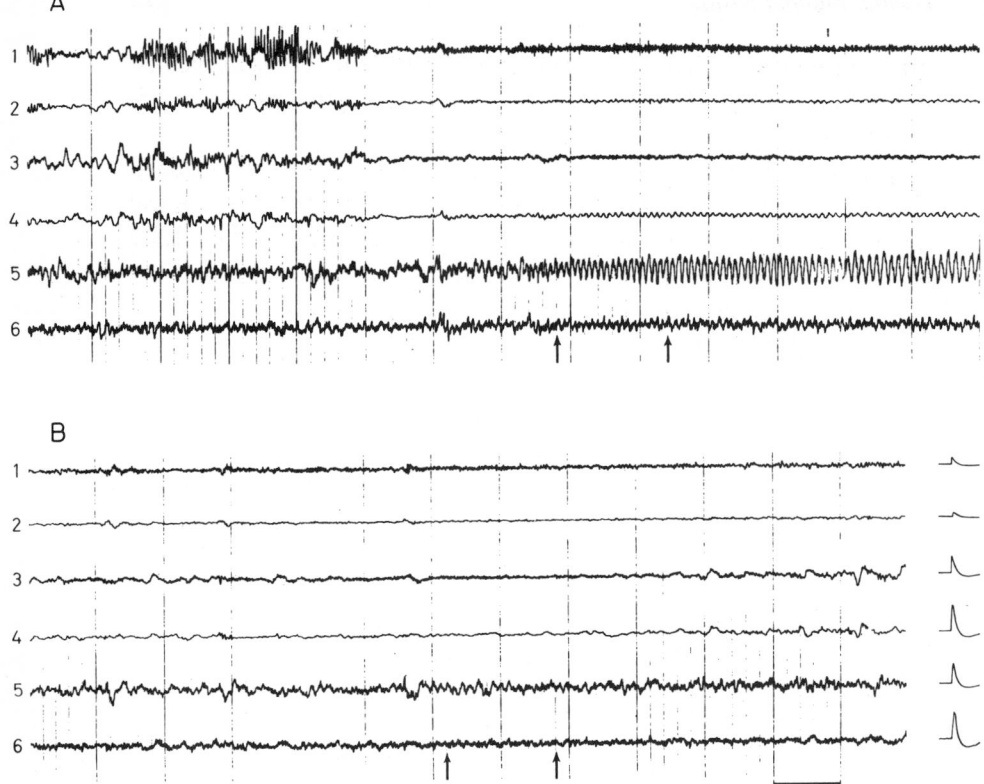

Figure 4.8
Effect of LSD on the cerebral electrical activity of the rabbit. In **A** are shown the resting and the arousal EEG patterns of the normal animal (*between the arrows*: acoustical stimulation). Note the theta waves in lead **5** (dorsal hippocampus) during arousal. Tracing **B** was registered 20 minutes after the i.v. administration of 50 μg/kg of the drug. The EEG is flattened and the stimulation does not modify the tracing. *Leads:* **(1)** L. anterior sensorimotor cortex; **(2)** L. posterior sensorimotor cortex; **(3)** R. posterior sensorimotor cortex; **(4)** L. optic cortex; **(5)** R. dorsal hippocampus; **(6)** mesencephalic reticular formation. Calibration: 2 sec., 100 μv.

(1966), amphetamine produces a similar effect on the "secondary" evoked cortical potential. The effect of LSD upon the electrical activity of the hippocampus of the rabbit seems more specific. Besides the disruption of the theta waves, LSD also causes the disappearance of the spontaneous bursts originating in the hippocampal pyramidal neurons, as demonstrated by Brücke et al. (1961) by means of microelectrode registration (Figure 4.9). A similar effect on the EEG and on the single-unit activity was described for tryp-

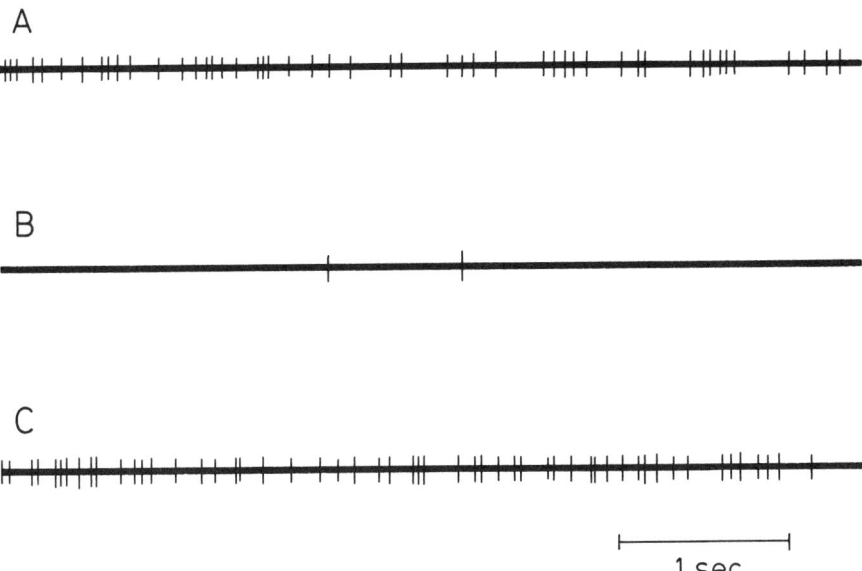

Figure 4.9
Effects of LSD on the electrical activity of a pyramidal hippocampal cell. **(A)** control tracing, registered in the curarized rabbit. **(B)** 5 minutes after i.v. administration of 100 μg/kg of the drug. The unit firing of the cell is almost abolished. **(C)** Recovery is observed 50 minutes later. (Modified, from Brücke et al., 1961.)

tamine (Baran et al., 1964); this further supports the theory that the central actions of LSD are probably dependent on a serotoninergic effect.

Knowing that LSD generally impairs intellectual processes in man (resulting in confusion, inappropriateness of action, and difficulty in thinking), researchers, have sought a counterpart of these effects in animals, specifically, in animals trained to perform various learned responses. The results of these investigations have indicated that the effect of LSD is observable only in complex situations. In rather simple tasks, like that of conditioned avoidance in rats, LSD does not have a striking effect; blocking was found only with 1.5 mg/kg (Cook and Weydley, 1957). The response latency to a tone (indicating water reward) is increased only after 0.1 mg/kg (Ray and Marrazzi, 1961).

The difference in the effect of LSD in trials of increasing com-

plexity performed upon the same animal species is clearly demonstrated in experiments carried out by Longo et al. When LSD (50–
100 μg/kg) is administered to rabbits trained to perform a simple
conditioned response (pulling a ring with the mouth upon the sound
of a buzzer in order to get food), an enhancement and a prolongation of the response is observed (Sadowski and Longo, 1962). When
a discrimination is introduced (i.e., when the animal is trained to dis-
criminate between a continuous sound that is followed by a reward,
and an intermittent sound that is not followed by a reward), the
drug disrupts the response at doses of 25 μg/kg (McGaugh et al.,
1963). Similar results have been obtained by Jarvik and Chorover
(1960) and by Fuster (1959). Fuster found that small doses (2–8
μg/kg) lowered the percentage of correct responses in a discrimination of briefly presented visual cues (associated with food rewards).
Jarvik and Chorover found that LSD impaired the performance of
monkeys in a delayed-alternation test at doses as low as 5 μg/kg.

In evaluating the effects of LSD on animals, particularly in
relation to the problem of recognizing a specific syndrome as a
counterpart of the psychotogenic action in man, careful consideration should be given to the fact that the metabolism of the drug
differs from species to species. In the first experiment on the distribution and fate of the drug in mice, C_{14}-labeled LSD was employed
(Stoll et al., 1955). The LSD disappeared rapidly from the blood
and was excreted by the liver and bile; only a very small fraction of
the dose was recovered from the brain and other organs, and the
major part of the unexcreted agent accumulated in the intestine in
the form of several metabolites closely related to LSD. The extremely rapid disappearance of the drug suggested that the psychic
changes were due more to a "trigger reaction" than to the presence
of the drug in the central nervous system (Haley and Rutschmann,
1957).

The development of exquisitely sensitive spectrofluorometric
methods subsequently permitted observation of the dynamics of the
fate of the drug. It could be shown that in man, LSD (2 μg/kg
intravenous) was present in the plasma for several hours after its
administration. In fact, a correlation has been noticed (Figure 4.10)
between the impairment of some psychic functions and the blood
level of the compound (Agajanian and Bing, 1964). The compari-

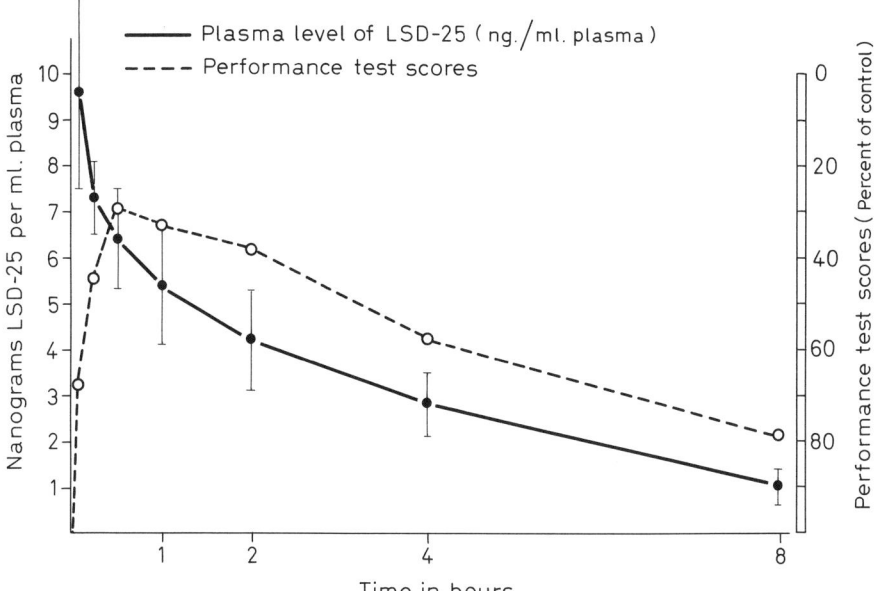

Figure 4.10
Relationships between LSD levels in plasma and effects on the brain. The *continuous* line indicates plasma levels after intravenous injection to an adult normal man of 2 μg/kg of LSD; the *broken* line indicated the performance ability expressed in test scores (from Aghajanian and Bing, 1964).

son of these data with those obtained in animals illustrates clearly the differences in metabolism among various species: the biological half-life of LSD in blood is respectively 7 minutes for mice, 100 minutes for monkeys and 175 minutes for man.

PSILOCYBIN

History

In their reports on the marvels of the new world, the Spanish chroniclers who followed the *conquistadores* frequently alluded to various preparations used by priests and witchdoctors during magical and divinatory ceremonies. In addition to herbs (such as ololiuqui) and cacti (such as peyote), mushrooms that produced "drunkenness, excitation, violence, and terror" were described. These ritually gathered mushrooms were called "teonanacatl" (God's flesh) and eaten raw for the purpose of achieving communion with the spirit world. Rituals of this type, modified in the course of the years separating us from the Cortesian period, are still in use in certain villages in southern Mexico, although they are seldom mentioned in the reports of modern ethnographers.

It is to the initiative of R. G. Wasson, a banker and a passionate amateur ethnographer, that we owe our knowledge of the use of these mushrooms. Searching for proof of the survival of the use of teonanacatl in religious rites, Wasson and his wife visited Central America in 1953. They were successful in locating and in gaining admittance to such rites; in the course of one, Wasson ingested mushrooms and underwent an hallucinatory experience.

Subsequently, expeditions by teams of specialists were organized, in which Professor R. Heim (the director of the Museum of Natural History in Paris) participated. As a result, various mushrooms used in the ceremonies were collected, identified, and cultivated in the laboratory. Isolation and identification of the active principles followed; these researches were carried out with the help of the investigators of the Sandoz Laboratories, who ultimately succeeded in synthetizing the active principles of the mushrooms. The documentation (Heim and Wasson, 1958) pertaining to this development reveals the brilliant interdisciplinary work that brought about the isolation of an indolic, structurally simple derivative, psilocin (Figure 4.11); this compound, a chemical relative of serotonin, proved to be responsible for the psychotomimetic effect that follows the ingestion of the mushroom. In nature, this substance is found either in its free form or coupled with a molecule of phosphoric acid. The latter compound, psilocybin, yields the active component upon ingestion.

The mushrooms that contain these substances belong to the genus *Psilocybe* and to the genus *Stropharia*. Some 15 varieties of *Psilocybe* were found to be capable of causing the psychotropic effect. *Psilocybe mexicana*, readily grown in the laboratory, was the main source of psilocybin before synthetic methods were developed. *P. mexicana* is a relatively small mushroom from 5-to-8 cm tall, with a dark-brown head 2 cm in diameter (Figure 4.12). In artificial cul-

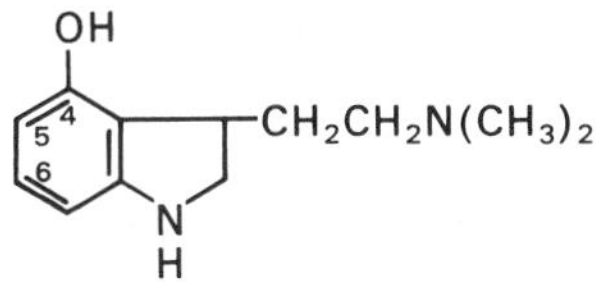

OH

$CH_2CH_2N(CH_3)_2$

Psilocin

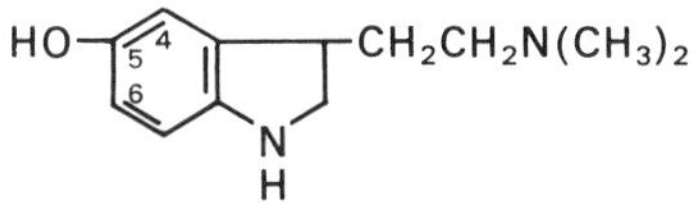

HO — $CH_2CH_2N(CH_3)_2$

Bufotenine

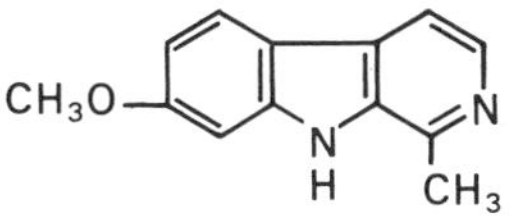

CH_3O —

Harmine

N
H CH_3

$CH_2CH_2N(CH_3)_2$

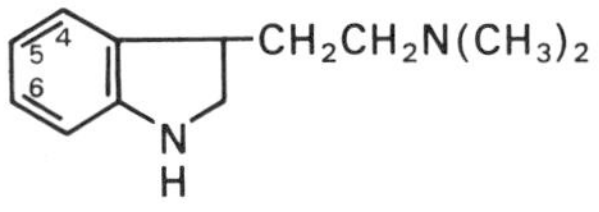

Dimethyltriptamine

Figure 4.11
Chemical formulas of some indole derivatives with psychotogenic action. Bufotenine
is an isomer of psilocin; the different positions of the hydroxyl group strongly influence the pharmacological actions of these two drugs. The side effects of bufotenine
are much more marked, and the drug is considered quite dangerous (see text).
Harmine, a β-carboline, can be considered a triptamine with the indole-ring side
chain cyclized.

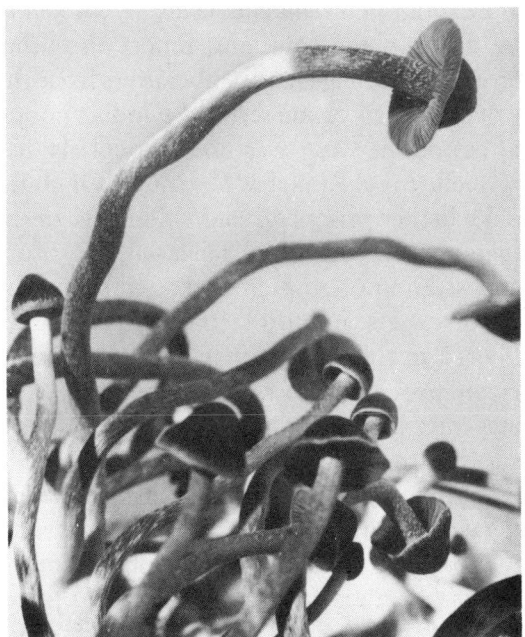

Figure 4.12
Psilocybe mexicana, Heim, grown in the laboratory.
A handful of these mushrooms, ingested raw, induces
the hallucinogenic experience. (Courtesy of A.
Hofmann, Basle.)

tures the mushroom tends to grow hypogeous tubercles, rich in active principles. Other species of *Psilocybe* that can induce hallucinations are the *P. semperviva, P. wassonii, P. aztecorum,* and *P. yungensis.*

Effects of the Mushroom and of Psilocybin on Man

Aside from the early Spanish chronicles and the folklore of the Indian tribes, the first detailed description of *Psilocybe* intoxication was given by Heim and Wasson (1958). This description was based on self-experiments as well as on observations of Indians under the influence of the preparation. These authors note the occurrence of somatic effects and of hallucinations and distortions of time and space—all of which are virtually the same as those produced by mescaline and LSD. In addition, Heim and Wasson, who emphasize the influence of the drug on the emotions, report an outburst of tender, generous, brotherly feelings, and a liberation from the shyness and repression that seem to characterize the Indian populations in question. This effect of the drug was not particularly noted in subsequent studies (Isbell, 1959, Rinkel et al., 1961). Of course, the question can be asked whether prisoners, paid volunteers, or psychopaths, on whom experiments are usually carried out, constitute ideal subjects for the demonstration of an increased affective resonance—and whether a hospital ward is an ideal setting for such an experiment. It should be noted in this respect that psilocybin has widely replaced LSD in private psychedelic sessions in the United States in recent years. Perhaps this increasing preference is related to the motivation for the use of the drug among the Indian populations.

Studies carried out in man have established that the somatic and psychic actions of psilocybin and psilocin are analogous to those of LSD and mescaline, although the duration of action is much shorter (2–4 hours). The cross-tolerance found between LSD, mescaline, and psilocybin suggests that these substances indeed possess some basic properties in common (Isbell et al. 1961). Effective doses in man vary between 5 and 15 mg, (orally or parenterally). Autonomic side actions precede the development of psychic symptoms. Thus, nausea, headache, and restlessness are common; mydriasis is always present; sometimes, rather than tachycardia and hypertension, a slight diminution of the cardiac rate and of the arterial blood pressure is observed.

Effects of Psilocybin on Animals

Studies of acute toxicity with psilocybin demonstrate that the latter does not exhibit the excitatory actions that are characteristic of LSD nor the convulsive effects that are observed following large doses of mescaline. In fact, in some animal species, such as the rabbit and the monkey, a clear-cut sedative action is observed. The rabbit does exhibit mydriasis, tachycardia, and hyperthermia, although these symptoms are not as marked as those observed after LSD. Blood-pressure effects are variable. In some animals, such as the cat, hypertensive action predominates; in others, such as the dog, hypotension is always obtained. Psilocybin enhances the spinal reflexes in the cat; by contrast, the indole derivatives with a substitution in position 5 have an opposite effect. The effect of psilocybin in isolated organs is not striking; psilocybin is a hundred times weaker than LSD in antagonizing the stimulating effects of serotonin in the rat uterus.

The effects of psilocybin on cerebral electrical activity are different from those of LSD, but rather resemble those of mescaline. While low doses (1 mg/kg) activate the EEG tracing, higher doses (3 mg/kg) induce the appearance of slow rhythms. As other hallucinatory drugs, psilocybin markedly affects the hippocampal theta waves of the rabbit; similarly, in the cat, there are EEG changes in the hippocampal system (Adey, 1964). Psilocybin interferes with learning, particularly when the task requires discrimination on the part of the animal (Adey et al., 1962; Baran and Longo, 1965).

MINOR HALLUCINOGENS

All the substances discussed so far induce in man a syndrome in which the distortion of perceptions (accompanied by illusions and hallucinations) predominates; additionally, side effects appear, which, however, are not marked. These substances may be considered as hallucinogens in the strict sense of the term. There are substances that produce psychomimetic and hallucinogenic effects only as a part of a general intoxication; therefore, their hallucinogenic effect is less specific. Some of them have been identified as present in various plants used for centuries in rituals and in folk medicine. Here belong substances such as harmine (known also as telepatine or banisterine), bufotenine, dimethyltryptamine; others, such as diethyltryptamine, have been synthetized in the laboratory. All these substances are indoles, and interesting hypotheses concerning the relationship between (1) hallucinogenic effect and (2) chemical structure were evolved on the basis of comparative studies on these compounds (Hofmann, 1968). It seems that a substitution in position 4 of the indole ring results in the hallucinatory syndrome with minimal side effects (Figure 4.11). It should be remembered that, among the specific hallucinogens, both LSD and psilocybin possess this special structural feature.

Bufotenine

As bufotenine is 5-hydroxydimethyltryptamine, it differs from psilocin only in the position of the hydroxylic radical (Figure 4.11). Originally isolated from the secretion of skin glands on the toad, it can be found also in various plants; its presence in the *Amanita muscaria* (see below) is doubtful. Certain tribes of the West Indies (Haiti) and of South America (Venezuela) have employed since pre-Colombian days a narcotic snuff prepared with the seeds of *Piptadenia peregrina*, a tree of the family of Leguminosae, related to the genera *Mimosa and Acacia*. The seeds are pulverized and mixed with lime and are insufflated into the nostril by means of Y-shaped tubes (Figure 4.13). The preparation is called "yopo," "paricà" or "epéna" by the South American populations and "cohoba" in the Greater Antilles. In ancient times, its use was as widespread as the use of tobacco snuff.

Because of the similarities in the tools and the methods employed in snuffing, the attempts of the ethnobotanists to classify and match the various preparations with the botanical sources were often frustrated. In recent years it has been demonstrated that *P. peregrina* is by no means the only source of the inebriating snuffs.

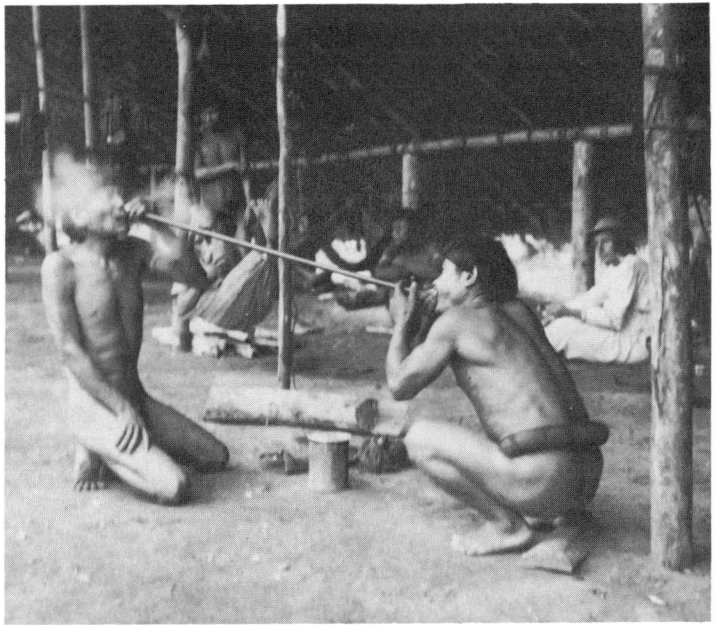

Figure 4.13
Ceremony of epena insufflation, photographed by George Seitz during his visit to the Waika ("Killer") tribes in the region of the upper Rio Negro, on the boundaries between Brazil and Venezuela (courtesy of the author).

According to Seitz (1967), for instance, paricà and epéna (snuffs that were believed to be prepared from the same botanical source as yopo) actually derive from a resin flowing from the bark of a tree, *Virola callophylloidea* (Myristicaceae). Holmstedt (1965) made an intensive investigation of the main constituents of six snuffs used by South American Indians, finding various amounts of tryptamine derivatives, in particular bufotenine, dimethyltryptamine and 5-methoxydimethyltryptamine. Mention is made in early reports of the use of these snuffs in religious and witchcraft rituals and before fights and hunts. In more recent times, however, Seitz (1967) was not able to identify any ritual reason for taking epéna, which now seems to be used rather as a voluptuary than as a transcendental drug.

The symptoms of intoxication following the nasal administration of all these compounds are very similar. Vasomotor and other neurovegetative phenomena are the first to appear and consist of headache, swelling and reddening of the face and extremities, intense perspiration, and vomiting. A period of excitation follows during which ataxia, yelling, tremors or even convulsions are observed. Finally, a state of stupor and sleep occurs. According to Becher (quoted by Holmsted, 1965) it seems that macropsia is the only symptom due to an effect of the preparation on the sensorium. There are no real hallucinations.

Several substances found in these various indigenous preparations were studied clinically and pharmacologically. The effects of bufotenine in man were investigated by Fabing and Hawkins (1956) at doses of 1–16 mg. They reported that bufotenine causes the appearance of color visions of an elementary character (spots, squares) and a certain feeling of relaxation and lightweightedness. Side effects were always predominant and very disturbing, and included nausea, vomiting, bronchospasm, and a purple hue of the skin resembling that associated with the vasomotor changes accompanying hyperserotoninemia due to carcinoid disease. Turner and Merlis (1959) obtained negative results with the powders of *Piptadenia* obtained from various sources, as well as with bufotenine and dimethyltryptamine, given to normal and schizophrenic subjects. Intranasal administration was effective only in provoking serious side effects; moreover, bufotenine, given parenterally, proved quite toxic, confirming unpublished data of Isbell, who later again called the attention to the dangerous cardiovascular effects of the drug (Isbell, 1967). The negative results obtained with bufotenine possibly could be explained by the fact that, in the case of the preparations employed by the Indians, the psychotomimetic effect may be due not to the action of a single component but to the combined effects, and possibly to the mutual potentiating action of the various indole derivatives present in the preparation.

Effects on Animals. Animal experiments demonstrate that the acute toxicity of bufotenine is greater than that of psilocybin, the somatic and autonomic effects being particularly marked. In the case of primates, relatively high doses of the substance (5 mg/kg, intravenous) induce a paralytic syndrome of short duration followed by catatonia and tameness (Evarts, 1958). Similarly, in other animals a motor deficit accompanied by serious autonomic disturbances was described (Rinaldi, 1958, Himwich et al., 1960). It should be added that the intensity of these side effects raises some doubts as to whether the effects of bufotenine on conditioned behavior (Baran and Longo, 1965) are due to the specific effect of the drug on the central nervous system.

Electrophysiological studies demonstrated an effect of the drug on the EEG that resembles that provoked by LSD, mainly with regard to its action on the hippocampal theta rhythm (Rinaldi, 1958, Baran and Longo, 1965). Evarts (1958) found that bufotenine (0.2 mg/kg, intracarotid injection) diminishes the postsynaptic evoked response registered at the lateral geniculate. This finding agrees with the data of Curtis and Davis (1962), who found that the drug, applied electrophoretically *in situ*, prevents lateral geniculate neurons from responding to volleys applied to the optic nerve. All these effects of bufotenine resemble those of LSD (see above). It is, however, difficult to accept the notion that the effects of these drugs on the optic pathways explain the visual disturbances observed in the course of human intoxication. In fact, the psychotomimetic action of LSD and related compounds in the human subject is induced by doses that are much lower than those employed in the aforementioned experiments in animals. It is nevertheless important to have found a central synapse or synapses sensitive to drugs that induce hallucinations in man, as it is possible that even the minute psychotomimetically active doses of these compounds could still be capable of causing subtle alterations in the response of certain neurons, thus affecting central sensory integration.

Dimethyltryptamine and Diethyltryptamine

Dimethyltryptamine (DMT) (Figure 4.11) and bufotenine constitute the two most important ingredients of cohoba, yopo, and related South American snuffs. It is possible that the various substances present in the snuff potentiate each other with regard to the confusional syndrome that follows inhalation of the powders. In any event, DMT, administered parenterally at relatively high doses (50–100 mg), induces a number of disturbances described in detail by Szara (1957) who experimented with the drug upon himself. Among these disturbances, the hallucinogenic component was preponderant, either with alterations in perception or with the occurrence of actual hallucinations. At the same time, autonomic disturbances and peculiar motor manifestations consisting of choreiform compulsive movements appeared. Euphoria was present throughout the period of intoxication, which lasted only one hour. Szara experienced similar effects with diethyltryptamine (DET), except that the state of elation was either less marked or substituted by anxiety. Oral doses of either drug up to 150 mg were ineffective. It should be mentioned here that in recent years the practice of smoking or inhaling the fumes of DMT-containing preparations or natural products has been fashionable among drug users.

When the effects obtained in humans with DMT, DET, and bufotenine are compared with those of LSD, certain differences become obvious, differences that could throw some light on the action of these drugs. The effect of the tryptamine derivatives has a rapid onset and a very short duration. The time difference between the appearance of the vegetative and psychic disturbances characteristic for LSD does not exist in the case of the other drugs, which produce these effects simultaneously. The extrapyramidal involvement is minimal with LSD; it is marked during the intoxication with DMT and DET. Finally, with the simpler indole derivatives, sensory disturbances mainly occur in the visual system; the LSD alterations are more widespread across the sensorium.

Harmine and Related Compounds

Harmine is an alkaloid with a β-carboline structure (Figure 4.11) isolated towards the end of the last century from the seeds of *Peganum harmala*. *Peganum* is a plant native to the Middle East, whose medical and psychotropic properties have been known for many centuries. The same active principle was found in an intoxicating drink still used in an area lying between the rain forests of South America and the Andes. Different vernacular names are used for this beverage: "ayahuasca" (Dead man's vine), "caapi," "yagè," "natem." All are infusions prepared from a tropical vine of the Malpighiaceae family, *Banisteriopsis caapi*.

Usually the infusion is prepared according to traditional rituals and is drunk in the course of festivals, initiations, and magic-therapeutic practices. These rituals, which have a public character, have been recorded on film by several expeditions, most recently by D. Taylor's expedition in 1966 (Taylor, 1967). Several descriptions of the effects of the preparation are available; these descriptions show marked differences, which may be due to the addition of tobacco extracts or the juices of other plants to the infusion prepared from *B. caapi*. The intoxication generally presents the following course: (1) vertigo and emesis, (2) psychomotor excitement, (3) somnolence. Either during the stage of excitement or during that of the subsequent depression, visions occur, mainly in the form of geometrical patterns. A vivid and interesting description of self-intoxication was made by a sophisticated addict and brilliant writer, W. Burroughs (Burroughs and Ginsberg, 1963). He ingested a high dose of yagè and experienced a peculiar scintillation of crude colors, vertigo, ataxia, numbness of the body; at the peak of the drug's action, convulsions appeared, terminated by the prompt self-administration of pentobarbital.

In addition to these β-carbolines, Poisson (1965) found a substantial amount of dimethyltryptamine in the leaves of *Banisteriopsis rusbyana*. It is interesting to know that the samples studied and identified botanically by Poisson were obtained in the course of actual preparations of the concoction; this preparation included mixing the leaves of *B. rusbyana* with pieces of the creeper *B. caapi*, the latter being rich in harmine. These and other similar observations (Holmsted, 1967; Hochstein and Paradies, 1957) indicate that during the preparation various principles were expressly included, probably to obtain an enhancement and potentiation of action.

There are relatively few reported observations in the literature regarding the effectiveness in man of the pure components of the *B. caapi*. Harmine was studied by Pennes and Hoch (1957) on mental, generally schizophrenic, patients (therefore, the value of their studies is limited, as it is known that the schizophrenics react in a special way to drugs of this type). In any event, these authors reported perceptual disturbances, impairment of contact, and delirious reactions. Visual hallucinations occurred only in a few subjects and only when the drugs was administered intravenously (200 mg). According to the observations of Naranjo (1967) it appears that harmaline (dihydroharmine) present in the extracts of *B. caapi* is probably responsible for the psychodysleptic state due to the infusion. Naranjo treated normal subjects with 1 mg/kg, intravenously, or 4 mg/kg, orally, of harmine, comparing its effects with that of mescaline. Psychic and physical symptoms appeared together shortly after the administration of harmaline; distortions of forms or alterations of sensory perceptions were exceptional in the treated subjects, who, on the other hand, experienced true hallucinations in vivid colors with their eyes closed. Concern with religious or philosophical problems and a desire to communicate was not prominent. The subjects tended to be withdrawn and intensely absorbed in their visions. Physical symptoms were present during the intoxication and consisted of paresthesia all over the body, followed by numbness, vomiting, and headache. In preliminary trials, made by the same authors, hallucinogenic properties were also found in tetrahydroharmine, 6-methoxyharmalan, and 6-methoxytetrahydroharman. McIsaac (1961) stated that this latter product is identical with adrenoglomerulotropine, which is present in pineal gland tissue. McIsaac suggests that a psychotic state could be produced by some β-carbolines endogenously produced through some "error" in normal body metabolism.

Effects on Animals. The first systematic study of the effects of harmine, harmaline, and of other β-carbolines on laboratory animals was done by Gunn (1935). Tremors, convulsions, and excitation characterized the toxic syndrome induced by harmine and harmaline. This has been confirmed by other investigators (Chen and Chen, 1939). Later on, an antimonoaminooxidase effect was attributed to harmine and harmaline as well as an antiserotonin action on smooth muscles (see Gyermek, 1966).

Other authors have in particular examined the effects of harmine on the central nervous system. Gershon and Lang (1962) reported a state of "anxiety" and excitation in the dog. Himwich et al. (1959) studied the effect of harmine on the cerebral electrical activity of the rabbit, describing EEG activation after the administration of 5 mg/kg. The tremorigenic effect of harmine in mice was analyzed by Hara and Kawamori (1954). These authors noticed that the tremors disappeared after ablation of either the cerebral cortex or striatum. On the basis of these findings, they suggested that the drug had an effect on the extrapyramidal system. Recent biochemical studies seem to uphold this theory; according to Poirier et al. (1968), harmaline has a specific effect on brain dopamine and hinders both its synthesis from L-DOPA and its conversion into homavanillic acid. Therefore, the tremor elicited by these alkaloids could be deemed analogous to the syndrome observed in mammals (monkeys) and man with lesions of the extrapyramidal system. This syndrome is antagonized by various centrally acting drugs such as the antiparkinsonians and antiepileptics. It is of interest to note also that LSD (0.25 mg/kg) is able to control harmine tremors (Zetler, 1957). As to the other derivatives with a β-carboline structure, literature dealing with pharmacological findings is scarce. Gunn points out that harmol causes a paralysis instead of the excitation observed with the methoxylated derivatives. The pharmacological properties of harmane were studied by Sigg et al. (1964); they described a convulsant effect.

The behavioral and electroencephalographic effects of harmine, harmaline, and five related β-carbolines (Figure 4.14) were studied by Fuentes and Longo (1971) in rats and rabbits bearing chronical-

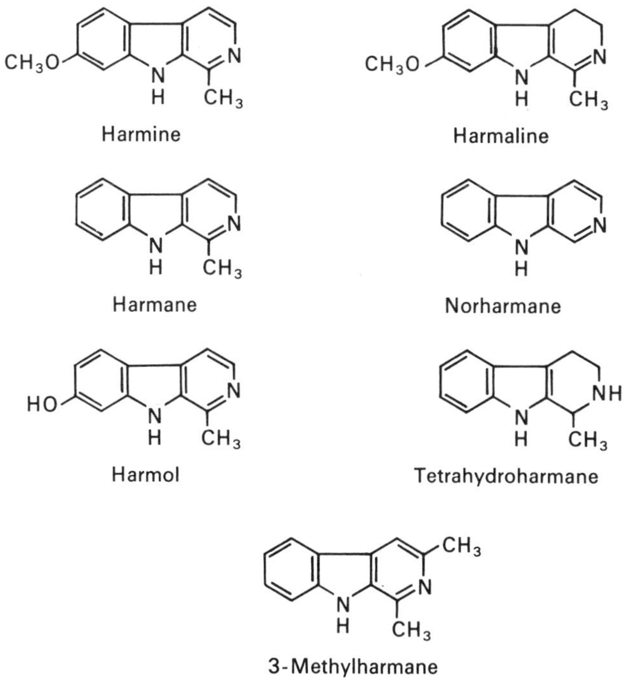

Harmine

Harmaline

Harmane

Norharmane

Harmol

Tetrahydroharmane

3-Methylharmane

Figure 4.14
Chemical formulas of harmine, harmaline, and other related β-carbolines. (For structure-activity relationships, see text.)

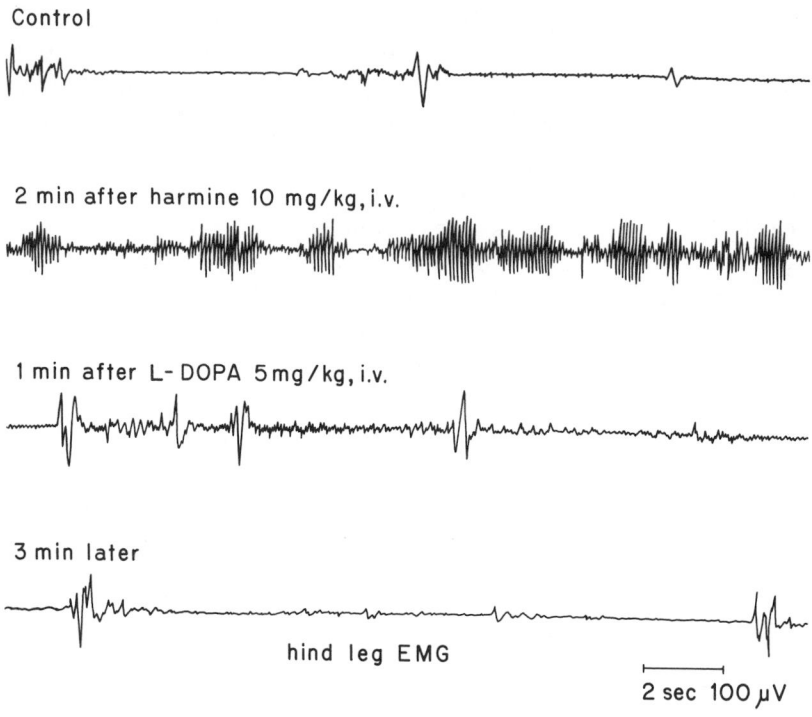

Figure 4.15
Antagonistic effect of L-DOPA on harmine tremors in the rabbit. A bipolar needle-electrode is inserted in the hind-leg muscles. After administration of harmine, the characteristic waxing and waning tremor appears, which disappears three minutes after administration of L-DOPA.

ly implanted electrodes in various cortical and subcortical areas. Based on the results obtained, the seven derivatives were divided into three groups. The first group includes harmine and harmaline, which caused excitation, tremors, and ataxia both in the rat and in the rabbit. The modification of the cerebral electrical activity during the tremors consisted of an increase in frequency and in voltage, observed in the cortical leads. Harmol, tetrahydroharmane, and 3-methylharmane caused a completely different toxic picture, consisting of a depressive syndrome, which can extend to complete paralysis in the rat. Harmane and norharmane produced, at low doses, a motor depression having a catatonic component; higher doses led to clonic and tonic-clonic type convulsions; tremors were never observed. In the rabbit, but not in the rat, L-DOPA was effective in antagonizing the tremors and the other toxic symptoms caused by the two drugs (Figure 4.15). These results suggested that the tremors induced by harmine and harmaline may be caused by an effect on the extrapyramidal dopaminergic system.

Ololiuqui

Ololiuqui is still another substance used by South American Indians as an intoxicant and hallucinogenic agent. The substance was described by the early Spanish chronicler Francisco Hernández, who gave us an accurate account of coaxihuitl (snake plant) and of its small, lentiform seeds, called ololiuqui (meaning "round object" in the local language). The drug is used ritually to *versare cum superis, ac reposta accipere ab eis* (communicate with the gods and receive the secret things from them).

For many years the botanical classification of the plant was debated; it was first classified correctly among the Convolvulaceae (morning glory) and subsequently among the Solanaceae, perhaps on the basis of Hernández's report, which described psychic effects of the plant similar to those observed in the course of atropine intoxication. Lewin, in his book Phantastica, refers to ololiuqui as a substance originating in *Datura meteloides*. Finally, Schultes (1941) recognized in a Convolvulacea, *Rivea corymbosa*, the source of ololiuqui. Much more recently, Wasson, who brought the seeds of ololiuqui from Central America, made it possible to grow two species of the plants belonging to the morning-glory variety, *Rivea corymbosa* and *Ipomoea violacea*. The identification of the active principles of the seeds was made by Hofmann and Tscherter (1960) and this led to the isolation of a series of lysergic-acid derivatives, which thus were obtained for the first time from a botanical source other than fungi (Figure 4.16). The seeds of *R. corymbosa* and of *I. violacea* contained 0.012 and 0.06 percent, respectively, of indole alkaloids.

Effects in Man. Inconsistencies and controversy characterized the study of the psychic effects of ololiuqui. We owe the first careful, detailed account of the effect of the ingestion of this substance to Osmond (1955), who reported the occurrence of a "strange mental

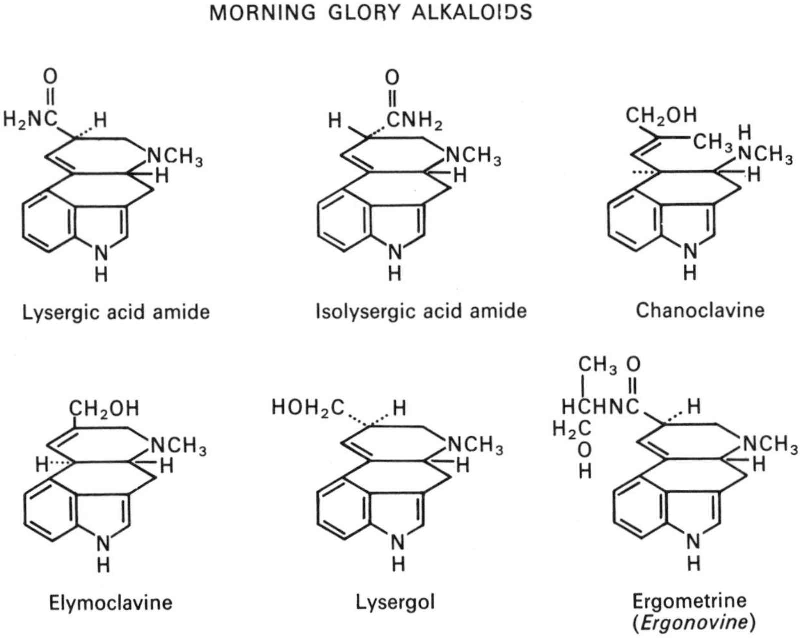

MORNING GLORY ALKALOIDS

Lysergic acid amide

Isolysergic acid amide

Chanoclavine

Elymoclavine

Lysergol

Ergometrine
(*Ergonovine*)

Figure 4.16
Alkaloids isolated from the seeds of *Ipomoea violacea* and *Rivea corymbosa* (morning-glory varieties). The occurrence of this type of chemical structure in higher plants is unusual. Lysergic acid amide was synthetized and tested in humans many years before its identification in these plants.

state" upon ingestion of 100 seeds of *R. corymbosa*. The seeds were ground to powder and swallowed with water. The reaction consisted of apathy, withdrawal, and sedation, with few or no visual symptoms or sensory distortions. A similar reaction was described by Hofmann and Cerletti (1961) who self-experimented with an extract of the seeds. On the other hand, negative results were reported by Kinross-Wright (1959).

When the various alkaloids of ololiuqui were isolated by Sandoz researchers, it was realized that one of the substances identified, the lysergic-acid amide, had been not only synthetized before but also used in a clinical study by Solms (1956) under the code name LA 111. Solms reported predominantly sedative properties and only a slight psychodysleptic effect. Although there is strong presumptive evidence indicating that the amide is the principal component responsible for the psychotropic action of ololiuqui, the final proof has still to be provided.

Perhaps in this case, as in that of other hallucinogenic preparations used by the Indians, only the mixture of various components provides an optimal psychotropic effect. Using this concept as a guideline, Isbell and Gorodetzky (1966) compared the effect of the extract with those of a mixture of six main constituents in their pure form, in the ratio in which they were present in the extract. Five milligrams of the extract and of the alkaloid mixture (corresponding in either case to about 400 seeds) were diluted in syrup and given orally to six healthy males, ex-opiate addicts. The effects of the crude extract and of the synthetic mixture were similar, but distinctly different from those of LSD. Symptoms observed with both mixtures were nausea, headache, increase in blood pressure, mydriasis, indifference, and sleepiness; hallucinations did not occur, and there were only a few reports of sensory distortions. Thus, controlled studies did not support the claim that ololiuqui possessed hallucinogenic and euphoric properties; the effects reported after ingestion of the seeds by maladjusted persons (Fink et al., 1966) could well be due to their suggestibility or to ingestion of other drugs. It should be added that the indiscriminate use of morning-glory seeds, which are commercially available, may be dangerous (Fink et al., 1966). Besides the symptoms already described, others may occur due to incorrect and sometimes incredible extracting and administering procedures (as for instance, intravenous self-injection of alcoholic extracts); there is also the potential danger of ergotism, which is particularly likely to occur if seeds are ingested repeatedly.

It should be noted that other substances are present in the ololiuqui seeds. For instance, the isolation and partial characterization of a glucoside has been described by Cook and Kieland (1962). This substance, administered to rabbits, proved fatal at a dose of 30 mg/kg.

Fly Agaric (Amanita Muscaria)

The mushrooms called fly agaric (*Amanita muscaria*) have long been used as an inebriant in northern Siberia, from the Ob river valley to the Kamchatka peninsula. Written reports that deal with

the use of this mushroom to produce temporary ecstatic states, depersonalization, and hallucinations date back as far as the eighteenth
century. Other reports were subsequently published, and Lewin in
his book *Phantastica* (1924) had an entire chapter on the agaric. All
these reports, however, seem to be based mainly on second-hand
information, often transmitted from the same source. It seems probable that ethnopharmacological research on this mushroom has been
recently carried out in Russia (Brekhman and Sam, 1967); if so,
however, the results have not been made widely available.

Wasson (1967) outlined certain characteristics of the intoxication, based also on self-experiments carried out by him and his
friends. He found that a few carpophores suffice to elicit psychic
effects. They can be ingested raw, their pressed juice can be drunk,
or they can be toasted and eaten with soup or other infusions. The
first phase of the effect, which ensues 15–20 minutes following ingestion, is that of depression and consists of a sleep-like state, during
which visions may be present. The second phase is one of elation and
excitement, accompanied by vivid imagery, distortions of sight, and
auditory hallucinations. The Siberians discovered that the urine of
an intoxicated person, if ingested, could provoke the hallucinatory
experience. This seems to be confirmed by recent experiments made
by Waser (1967) who ingested some active principles of the
Amanita muscaria and then found in his urine a substance that was
chemically similar to the ingested compound.

There are still doubts as to whether the ancient inhabitants of
Scandinavia were using the same mushroom for becoming euphoric
and aggressive before battles. The "berserk rage" of the ancient
Scandinavian warrior consisted of shivering, tremors, reddening of
the face, cries, and incoordinate movements. In view of what is
known of similar events in other populations, in which the use of
related drugs was transmitted from generation to generation, it is
surprising that there is no mention in Scandinavian mythology or
sagas of the use of inebriating substances, whether identical with fly
agaric or, for that matter, completely different.

The Hallucinogenic Principles of Amanita Muscaria. *Amanita muscaria* is indigenous to most of Europe, and it also grows in North
America. Its accidental ingestion frequently induces intoxication,
sometimes serious but rarely fatal (Buck, 1963). The studies of the

active principles present in the mushroom were initiated more than 100 years ago. Muscarine, a powerful parasympathomimetic substance, was thus identified; among other substances found in the mushroom were choline, acetylcholine, atropine, hyoscyamine, and bufotenine. While the three last substances are hallucinogenic, they are present in the mushroom in such small quantities that they could not be responsible for the psychic syndrome that follows the ingestion of *Amanita muscaria*. After a number of studies, it was concluded that the inebriating effect was due to an unidentified substance, called pilzatropine.

The isolation of the hallucinogenic principle came from an unexpected lead. The name of the *Amanita muscaria* accounts for the reputation of this mushroom as a fly and a bug poison. After recognition of the structure of muscarine (Kögl et al., 1957; Eugster et al., 1958), Swiss investigators at the University of Zürich, continued to search for other active substances, supported by funds from Geigy. Apparently, the search was successful in isolating some pure substances, but the results were not made public, probably because of commercial implications. In 1964, Japanese investigators reported the isolations from *Amanita pantherina* of three fly-killing crystalline substances, giving also the correct structure for two of them, ibotenic acid and pantherine.

Later on, other works were published by English and Swiss investigators, which, although using a different terminology, showed the same structures as described by the Japanese (Figure 4.17). In addition to pantherine (agarin, muscimol) and ibotenic acid, a third constituent was described by Eugster, and called muscazone (see, for references, Eugster, 1967). In the papers of the latter authors, emphasis was placed not on fly-killing properties, but on the narcotic potentiation shown by the substances. Muscimol and ibotenic acid were studied pharmacologically and were found to affect the brain in a selective manner; i.e., they seem devoid of peripheral effect. Typical signs of intoxication are excitation, dilated pupils, cramps, and hyperpnea, followed by sedation. Muscimol exhibits a pronounced sedative effect, and potentiates the narcosis produced by other hypnotics. Other indications of a central effect are a certain antiemetic and antitussive property and the EEG changes observed in rabbits and cats. At small doses (0.5 mg/kg), a synchronizing effect is noted, with the appearance of slow waves in the tracing. At

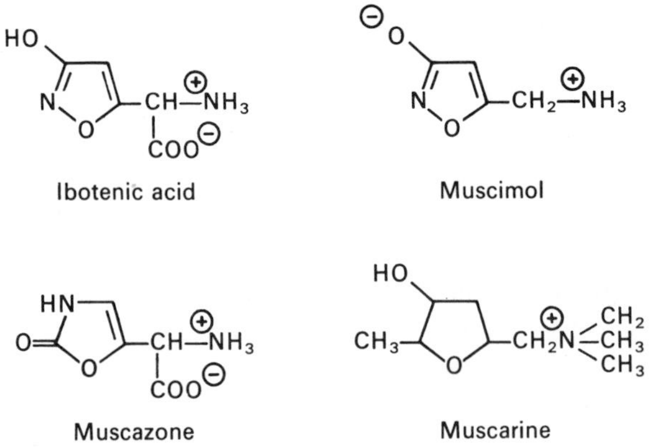

Figure 4.17
Chemical structures of muscimol, ibotenic acid, and muscazone, compared with that of muscarine; all these substances are present in *Amanita muscaria*. While ibotenic acid is found in the mushroom in considerable quantities (up to 1 g per kg of fresh carpophores), the content of muscarine is much lower (0.0002%). According to Eugster (1967), ibotenic acid acts as a precursor for both muscimol and muscazone. Probably, in the mushroom there are other active substances, the structures of which are not yet identified.

high doses (2–5 mg/kg), muscimol provokes the appearance of spikes (Theobald et al., 1968).

Reporting on self-experiments, Waser (1967) points out that 10–15 mg of muscimol, orally, produces a toxic psychosis with confusion, myoclonic jerks, and disturbances of visual perceptions ("echo picture"), followed by fatigue and sleep. Ibotenic acid was devoid of psychic effects when given in doses of up to 20 mg. Further experiments (Theobald et al., 1968) have shown that the syndrome obtained with muscimol hardly compares with that due to LSD or psilocybin, but rather resembles an acute exogenous reaction. However, a more detailed investigation on the effects in man of the substances extracted from *Amanita muscaria* is highly desirable. For example, it would be interesting to study the effects of various combinations of muscimol, ibotenic acid, and muscazone given together, for such a mixture would be present when the mushroom itself is ingested.

Indian Hemp (Hashish, Marihuana)

Indian hemp *(Cannabis indica)* is a variety of the species *Cannabis sativa*, a domesticated plant of great importance for the manufacture of cord, twine, and textiles. The diverse varieties of hemp are known since antiquity not only for their commercial uses but also for the intoxicating properties of the ingredients present in the flowering tops (including flowers, leaves, and stems) of the feminine plants. Herodotus informs us that the Scythians burned hemp on charcoal and inhaled the fumes. It is also documented that the Chinese and Indians utilized the plants for voluptuary purposes. Pliny the Elder records this particular use. On the other hand, we find many references to the limitations of the use of hemp by law, beginning with the edicts of the emirs against its abuse in Arabia (in the 14th century) and continuing with its ban during the French occupation of Egypt in the first years of the 19th century. After a timid appearance in the pharmacopeias of various countries, accompanied by vague therapeutic indications, cannabis is listed today among substances subject to international control as a source of preparations that induce habituation and psychic dependence.

In Europe, the use of cannabis as a voluptuary agent was initiated in 1800; in the United States, the substance was introduced later, where it was imported from Mexico, under the name of marihuana or marijuana. The active substance (known as "hashish" or "kif" in North Africa; "maconha" in South America), is usually smoked in pipes or rolled in paper; sometimes it is mixed with tobacco. Taken in this way, it is mainly absorbed by the respiratory passages. However, oral preparations are also available. The plant material is mixed with sugar and flour, forming an electuary paste. It is also put in a drink with an alcoholic content. The ingestion of cannabis is particularly common in India, where the use of the chopped, dried material is not prohibited by the law. On the illegal market, the substance is available in two forms: the most common form is compressed packs of the flowers, leaves, and stems; solid bricks are prepared from the resin excreted by the flowers at a certain period, collected by such means as rubbing the tops of the plant by hand or with a piece of cloth. The resin can also be collected from the leather aprons of plantation workers who thrash their way among the plants. This resin contains a concentrate of the active agents and is therefore much more active than the botanical preparation.

Effects on Man. The effects of hemp have been described in many literary accounts as well as in many scientific reports. Charles Baudelaire (1860), Théophile Gautier (1846), and William Burroughs have written in detail of the experience of hashish inebriation. In the scientific realm, pharmacologists, chemists, and medical men engaged in research have reported on their subjective experiences with the drug. The psychiatrists Kant and Krapf (1928) provide a particularly masterful description on the effect of hashish upon themselves.

The symptoms of intoxication appear after a variable latency, which, among other factors, depends on the route of administration, being shorter upon inhalation than upon ingestion. The subject experiences first a feeling of well-being, improved ideation, and a facilitation of motor activity. Soon, however, the sense and the realization of time and space are lost and a torpor ensues. At this stage of the intoxication there is a flight of thoughts, visions, and a strange and pleasant sensation of swimming or flying. (These phenomena may be due to the loss of extero- and proprio-ception; painful sensations are also obtunded. Consciousness, however, is maintained in the main; the subject continues responding to queries, and he may be roused from the torpor.) Experiences of this sort may have given rise to the creation of fantastic personages, like the man on the flying carpet and the witch on the flying broomstick, widely illustrated through the centuries in popular iconography (Figure 4.18).

It should be stressed that individuals vary greatly in their reactions to the drug; moreover, the conditions under which the drug is taken differ greatly from society to society. In the East, hashish is smoked or drunk, and the devotee prefers to keep by himself, aiming particularly at the experiences connected with the second phase of intoxication. He remains seated or reclining, lost in his dreams. In the Western world, marihuana is a social drug, and the takers get together to smoke cigarettes (reefers) made with the flowering tops of cannabis. The inhalation of the drug is not devoid of secondary consequences. In order to achieve an effect, the smoke must be deeply inhaled; this leads to irritation of the respiratory passages, and

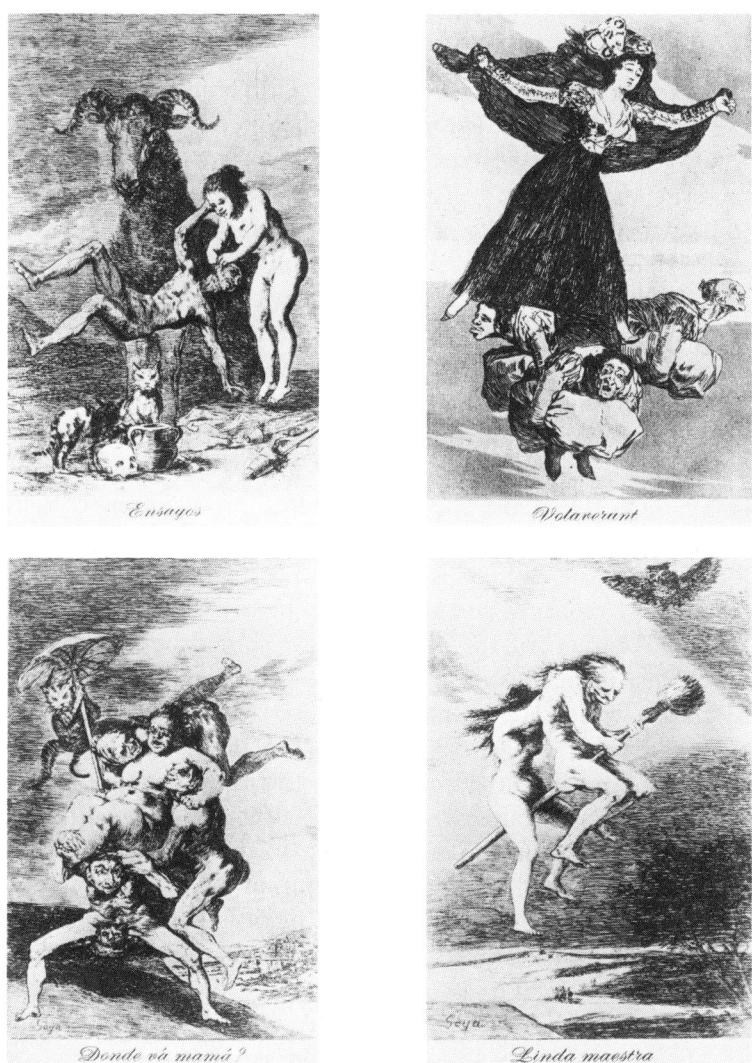

Figure 4.18
The theme of flight is common in the witchcraft section of Goya's engravings "Caprichos." Goya (1746–1828) was from the Basque provinces, where witchcraft has long been practiced. Goya intellectually rejected the supernatural; he felt that monsters and related phenomena originate only in distorted minds. His particular genius in drawing the products of his own imagination makes him a precursor of the investigation on perversions and the exploration of the subconscious.

In *Ensayos* (Attempts), the nude and levitating witch helps the initiate in his attempts to soar in the air; behind him looms a gigantic ram, clearly an hallucinatory figure. In the other engravings, *Volaverunt* (And they flew away), *Onde va mama?* (Where goes mother?), and *Linda Maestra* (Beautiful teacher) other flight modalities are poignantly illustrated.

may lead to bronchial spasms, coughing, and vomiting. It is difficult to say, in these sessions, to what extent the effect is due to the drug or to suggestion; in any event, there is soon improvement in affect, a characteristic inclination for comedy, a tendency to laugh or giggle. The participants move in a bizarre fashion as they follow their illusions; they are frequently hungry and sexually aroused. The sensation of hunger is particularly prominent after the drug effect is over, which is specific for this intoxication and distinct from the hangover which follows alcoholic intoxications.

Even though there is no general agreement on this question, it appears that tolerance to hashish is not marked; in fact, in the course of prolonged use the drug always induces similar psychic and organic effects. The most important medical problem related to the use of hashish is that of its chronic intake. In the Orient, where the use of hemp is moderate, it is considered to be a voluptuary agent not dissimilar to tobacco and alcohol; frequently, the use of the drug is associated with chronic delinquency; it should be kept in mind however, that in these countries the takers of hemp belong to lower social classes, which are naturally characterized by high unemployment, vagrancy, and legal delinquency. The problem is different in the United States and in Europe, where the use of hemp is popular among prosperous groups who take the drug for motivations and purposes different from those prevailing in the Oriental countries. The major medical risk of the use of hemp in the Western world is not so much related to acute intoxication (although an overdosage of the drug can cause anxiety, fear, and depersonalization) or subsequent excessive intake, as to the tendency of some habitués to resort to more active and dangerous drugs, such as morphine and heroin. In fact, hemp itself does not produce physical dependence. Antisocial behavior under the influence of the drug is frequently described but always depends on the predisposition and the character of the subject, his motivations and mood. Actual craving for the drug is minor compared to that of alcoholics and chronic smokers. A frequent observation, made particularly in India, correlates the use of hemp with the period of greatest sexual activity in man, so that frequently the drug, which has been used since adolescence, is spontaneously abandoned after the age of forty.

The Active Principles of Cannabis. A viscous reddish oil ("red oil") containing the active principles can be obtained by treating the resin

NATURAL CANNABINOIDS

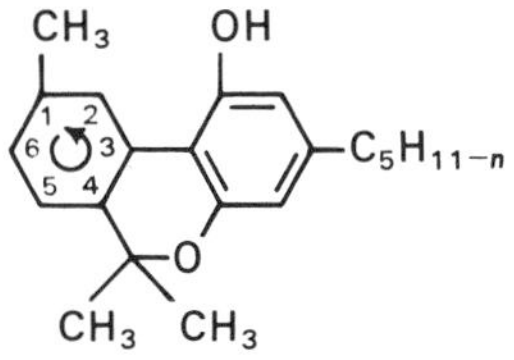

Isomeric
tetrahydrocannabinols

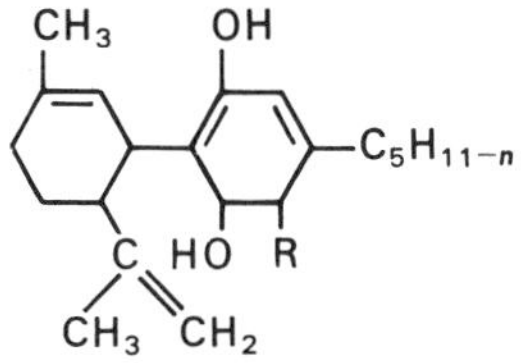

R = H : Cannabidiol
R = COOH : Cannabidiolic acid

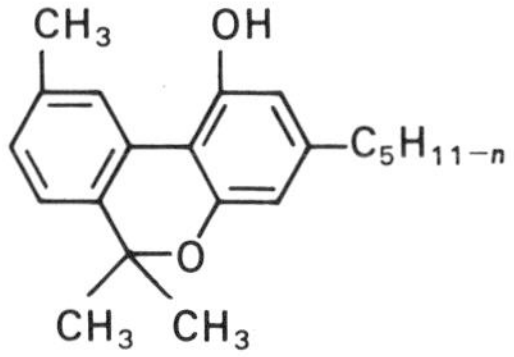

Cannabinol

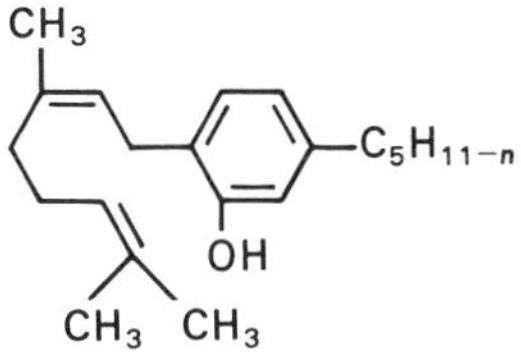

Cannabigerol

Figure 4.19
These compounds can be isolated from the "red oil" of cannabis.
Note that nitrogen is absent from their structures; therefore, these
substances cannot be classified as alkaloids. The euphoric and
hallucinogenic action of the oil should be attributed to the two
isomeric forms of tetrahydrocannabinol.

of the plant with organic solvents. Towards the end of the last century a "purified red oil" was obtained by distillation, which was inappropriately called cannabinol. Only much later was it proved that the "purified red oil" was actually a mixture of several chemically identifiable compounds: cannabinol, cannabidiol, and tetrahydrocannabinol (Figure 4.19). Subsequent investigations demonstrated the presence of two other components, cannabidiolic acid and cannabigerol (see, for references, Downing, 1962; Hofmann, 1968). American chemists (Adams, 1942) have moreover prepared a number of synthetic analogs of tetrahydrocannabinol; in the case of the synthetics, the *n*-penthylic side group of the mother

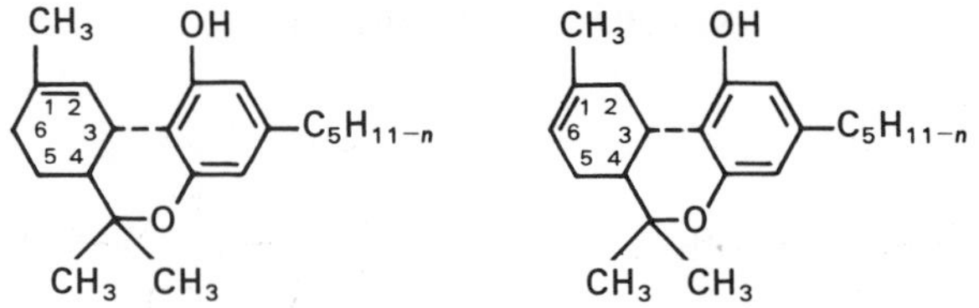

Δ^{1-2} (Δ^9) and Δ^{1-6} (Δ^8) Trans-tetrahydrocannabinol

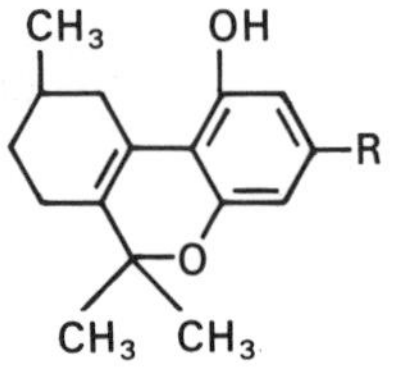

Synthetic compounds

DMHP: R = 1,2 dimethylheptyl
Synhexyl: R = *n*-hexyl

Figure 4.20
The racemic and levorotatory forms of the trans-tetrahydrocanna-
binols have been synthesized in the laboratory. Other synthetic
compounds, such as DMHP and Synhexyl have been studied both
in the laboratory and in the clinic.

substance was substituted by chains of various lengths as well as by
branching chains. The hexyl derivative (Parahexyl, Synhexyl) was
actually used in clinics as a stimulant and antidepressant (Figure
4.20). The most active synthetic was the 1,2-dimethylheptyl derivative (DMHP), which was studied pharmacologically rather extensively (see below).

The experiments on man and animals carried out with the
natural substances proved that the product most active centrally was
tetrahydrocannabinol, more precisely, an oil mixture containing a
number of isomeric forms of tetrahydrocannabinol (Loewe, 1950).
Cannabinol was slightly active, and the other products were devoid
of central action, although cannabidiolic acid was found to be
bacteriostatic (Kabelìk et al., 1960). This is not a surprising finding
as many earlier authors, including Rabelais, mention the antiputrefactive action of the plant extracts. The herb "pantagruelion,"

described by this author in the third book of *Pantagruel,* is none other than cannabis.

The relative content of the various substances in the resin is variable. It appears that in the course of the maturation of the plant, the psychically inactive cannabidiolic acid is transformed into tetrahydrocannabinol (Grlic and Andrec, 1961). Moreover, it is possible that, when smoked, the inactive components are transformed by the heat into active substances (Korte and Sieper, 1965). Similar transformations may occur when cannabis in ingested. Therefore, the extraction and identification of the components may have little relation to its pharmacological action. For these reasons, also, the standardization studies and biological studies encountered difficulties.

The precise position of the double bond in the molecule of tetrahydrocannabinol was only recently identified (see Hofmann, 1968). These researches also led to the synthesis of various compounds, among them $\Delta^{1-6}(\Delta^8)$- and $\Delta^{1-2}(\Delta^9)$-trans-tetrahydrocannabinol (THC); the spatial configuration and optical activity of these compounds was clearly established (Figure 4.20). Isbell et al. (1967) described the hallucinogenic and psychodysleptic activity of Δ^9-THC administered orally or by inhalation. This effect was similar to that of the extract of cannabis. Today the psychic effect of cannabis is ascribed to Δ^9-THC and to Δ^8-THC, always accepting the fact that some inactive substances present in cannabis can be transformed in the process of smoking or by biotransformation following ingestion.

Effects on Animals. The extracts of cannabis cause a characteristic intoxication in animals. These actions differ from those described for other hallucinogens; in its complexity, the syndrome partakes of the effects of a number of centrally active agents. The intoxicated animals exhibit both depressant and excitatory effects; although there is an increase of spontaneous activity, this increase is hindered in part by the motor deficit; the animals run around swaying and falling on their side, as described in the first pharmacological experiments carried out more than one hundred years ago by Liataud (1844). The "ataxic" action is one of the characteristic effects of the drug, and, while particularly evident in the dog, can also be obtained in other animals. Other symptoms are analgesia and corneal areflexia. Another illustration of the complex actions of cannabis is that it potentiates both the depressant action of the barbiturates and the excitatory action of amphetamine (Garriott et al., 1967).

Various bioassays have been proposed for the evaluation of the action of cannabis; the most frequently used are the ataxia test in the dog, developed by Loewe (1950), and corneal areflexia in the rabbit, developed by Gayer (1928). The analgesic action, although very marked, cannot be used for this purpose, as this action is common for many agents besides cannabis, including morphine and related compounds. It should be added that, generally, the natural substances were not studied in depth, so that very little data is available on the mechanism of action of these drugs. Perhaps the fact that researchers had to deal with a mixture rather than with a pure substance acted as a deterrent for more detailed studies. One of the most thoroughly studied substances, the synthetic dimethylheptylpyrane or DMHP (see before), is also a mixture of several isomers. Among other actions, DMHP depresses the polysynaptic spinal and supraspinal reflexes. This effect, similar to that of centrally acting muscle relaxants such as mephenesin, could explain the ataxic action of substances of this type. DMHP also produces a synchronization of the EEG in the cat and the attenuation of behavioral arousal and EEG arousal following the electrical stimulation of the reticular substance. These effects resembled those of pentobarbital (Dagirmanjian and Boyd, 1962; Boyd and Meritt, 1965). DMHP was also studied on various types of conditioned operant behavior; the drug depressed almost all of these behaviors in rats at a dose of 0.1 mg/kg (Boyd et al., 1963).

The more recent experiments, carried out with pure compounds such as Δ^9-THC or Δ^8-THC (Figure 4.20), demonstrated that the characteristic action of cannabis, that is, the ataxic, the analgesic, and the corneal effect, are obtainable with the pure agents (see, for references, Lipparini et al., 1969). In addition, evidence of hallucinatory behavior was obtained in cats and monkeys treated with the drugs; complex behavior involving memory or discrimination was markedly disrupted in monkeys, rabbits, and cats at doses as low as 2 mg/kg. Registration of the cerebral electrical activity in rabbits with chronically implanted electrodes showed that the levorotatory Δ^9-THC and Δ^8-THC produced a flattening of the tracing and a disappearance of the theta waves of the hippocampus very similar to that observed after LSD. Later on, spike-and-waves appeared in the tracings.

At present, the limitation due to lack of chemical identification is not a hindrance to experimentation, and the field is both open and promising for studies in depth of the effects of these substances. It is particularly interesting that the basic structure of the active components of cannabis is widely different from those of other hallucinatory agents; moreover, as it does not seem at present to be related chemically to the known transmitters, the elucidation of the mechanism of action of these drugs is challenging. This basic research should also throw light on the many obscure points concerning the human use of these drugs.

ANTICHOLINERGIC HALLUCINOGENICS

In the literature dealing with anticholinergic drugs, repeated mention is made of the central effects produced by the administration of these substances to man and animals. The prototypes of the anticholinergic substances are the alkaloids of the Solanaceae plants, atropine and scopolamine. Several analogs have been synthetized, some of which share with the natural alkaloids the property of antagonizing the effects of acetylcholine both at the peripheral and the central nervous system. The psychotomimetic effects of atropine and scopolamine have been known for a long time. Extracts of *Atropa belladonna, Hyoscyamus niger, Datura stramonium, Scopolia japonica, Duboisia myoporoides,* have been used as poisons and mind-altering drugs since the beginning of recorded history. Besides being used intentionally, these plants frequently cause accidental intoxications, since they are native to most of the world, and grow wild everywhere. The folklore names that one encounters clearly indicate that fatal or nearly fatal experiences with these plants are frequent. For instance, the red berries of *Atropa belladonna,* frequently ingested by children, are called "Tollkirsche" in Germany and "morella furiosa" in Italy. Herodotus recounted that the soldiers of Marcus Antonius became intoxicated in the course of a campaign in the Middle East when, during a period of famine, they ate a local plant, which was most likely *Datura stramonium.* During the state of confusion they incessantly overturned the stones and the rocks in the camp. The leaves of *Duboisia,* native of Australia and New Caledonia, are used to prepare an inebriating beverage. In the Middle East, other brain-affecting substances such as hemp or poppy seeds are sometimes "fortified" with a *Datura* extract. At the present time, youngsters of the Western World searching for thrills and excitement smoke a powder made up of *stramonium and belladonna* leaves, which in some places is available without prescription for the relief of asthma.

Peripheral and central symptoms overlap during intoxication with anticholinergic drugs, giving rise to a complex syndrome. Tachycardia, dryness of the mouth, mydriasis, and disturbances of accommodation that lead to blurred vision are present; in addition, profound behavioral and psychic disturbances, which are the central signs of intoxication, are also observed. These effects consist of impairment of memory, slurred speech, drowsiness, impaired motor ability, confusion and disorientation, unpleasant feelings, and hallucinations. After high doses, coma ensues. Although all the symptoms may appear alarming, death is rare, and usually the patient recovers even from coma, like Juliet in the Shakespeare drama, who awoke several days after drinking a draught of a potion made from belladonna leaves.

Central effects in many ways similar to those of atropine and scopolamine were also observed for other anticholinergic drugs. Table 4.2 sets forth some compounds that provoke transient psychopathological states in man. In the case of atropine and scopolamine, only a few references are quoted out of the many available in the literature. The exhaustive monograph of De Boor (1956), who reviewed the psychic and neurological syndrome produced by these drugs should be consulted. The works of Forrer (1951) and of Miller (1956), who used large doses (30–200 mg) of atropine and scopolamine for a sort of shock therapy ("atropine toxicity therapy") in some mental diseases are not noteworthy for their therapeutic effects but rather for their accurate description of the progress of the intoxication. Intoxication begins with a restless phase and continues through phases of muscular incoordination, disorien-

Table 4.2 *Psychotomimetic Effects of Anticholinergic Drugs on Humans*

Compound	Dose and Route	References
Atropine	32–200 mg, s.c.	De Boor, 1956; Forrer, 1951; Miller, 1956
Scopolamine	2.0 mg, oral	Ostfeld and Aruguete, 1962; Pfeiffer, 1959
Benactyzine	15–25 mg, oral 5–12 mg, s.c.	Vojtechovsky et al., 1968; Hess and Jacobsen, 1957
Trihexyphenydil	10 mg, oral	Pfeiffer, 1959
Caramiphen	25 mg, oral	De Boor, 1956; Pfeiffer, 1959
Adiphenine	100 mg, s.c.	Anichkov, 1959
Ditran	10–20 mg, oral and s.c. 2–5 mg, i.m.	Flügel and Itil, 1962; Abood, 1968
Ba 1433 (WH 4849)	5–15 mg, oral 20 mg, i.m.	Flügel and Bente, 1961; Flügel and Itil, 1962
AHR 376	2–4 mg, oral	Bente et al., 1964
Ro 2.3202/2	4 mg, s.c.	Schallek and Smith, 1952
Win 2299	2–10 mg, oral 2–5 mg, i.v.	Pennes and Hoch, 1957; Fink, 1960
7360 RP	25–75 mg, oral 50–200 mg, i.m.	Lambert et al., 1961
Hexamid	20–100 mg, i.v.	Flügel and Itil, 1962

tation, hallucinations, and, finally, coma. An important observation of these authors deals with the antidotal action of eserine. Irrespective of the amount of atropine used to produce coma, the intramuscular injection of 4 mg of eserine restored the patient's pretreatment status within a few minutes. This recovery, however, was transitory, and the patient became comatose again unless more eserine was given.

The other drugs listed in the table are all compounds that demonstrated atropine-like activities in the laboratory and were introduced in the clinic with various therapeutic connotations (sedatives, antiparkinsonians, spasmolytics). Some of these compounds had to be excluded from clinical use because of the seriousness of the psychic side effects but are still being used for experimental investigations of brain functions. Others are still employed clinically since side effects appear rarely and usually only with amounts significantly higher than the therapeutic doses. It should be considered, however, that in sensitive subjects a serious intoxication may appear even following mere instillation of a mydriatic anticholinergic into the conjunctival sac, and that all the "antiparkinsonian" drugs produce some degree of mental disturbance. This is particularly evident in parkinsonian patients who require for their activity complex higher integrative functions, for instance, executives or scientists.

Comparing the symptoms produced by these various compounds, it should be noticed that, within the range of a common syndrome, the different symptoms may vary in intensity, forming particular patterns for each individual drug. Scopolamine, for instance, seems to be a more potent sedative than the other compounds and more readily causes loss of recent memory and/or of the power of concentration; delirium and hallucinations are predominantly seen after benactyzine or the piperidyl benzylates (Ditran and analogs). The transient psychopathological conditions produced by these drugs present many similarities to symptoms seen in schizophrenia (see Abood, 1968). On the other hand, Vojtechovsky et al. (1968), who studied benactyzine in particular, have considered the confusion, the spatio-temporal disorientation, and the psychomotor stimulation as more akin to a delirium.

Several investigations have compared this syndrome with another type of "exogenous psychosis," that caused by LSD and related drugs. Even though some similarities between the two syndromes have been found (Pfeiffer, 1959), the majority of authors demonstrated that the two "psychoses" differ to a great degree (Isbell et al., 1964; Itil and Fink, 1968). The confusional picture following the anticholinergic drugs is always accompanied by a diminution of alertness and isolation from the environment, while LSD often elicits an extrovertive attitude. The anticholinergics provoke an apprehensive and anxious mood, which by no means can be compared with the "psychedelic" experiences obtained with LSD. An extensive discussion of these and other difference can be found in the review of Cerletti et al. (1963); Table 4.3, taken from this paper, summarizes the differences between the psychosomatic symptoms produced by LSD on the one hand, and those produced by the piperidyl benzylates on the other. It should be pointed out that the effects of other anticholinergics have many points in common with those elicited by the piperidyl benzylates.

The question arises whether all these manifestations can be

Table 4-3 *Differences in the Effects of Psychotomimetic Drugs Belonging to the Anticholinergic and to the Indole Group*

Piperidyl Benzilates	LSD, Mescaline, Psilocybine
Effects due to the block of the parasympathetic system: mydriasis, xerostomia, tachycardia, vasodilatation of skin capillaries	Effects due to stimulation of sympathetic system, mydriasis, tachycardia, hyperthermia
Slight influence on reflexes	Motor hyperreflexia
Apprehensive and anxious mood	Euphoria, pleasant feelings
Misinterpretation and isolation from the environment, tendency to introversion	Extrovertive attitude facilitating psychotherapeutic procedures
Predominantly auditory hallucinations	Predominantly visual hallucinations (kaleidoscopic)
Depersonalization only with high doses	Depersonalization commonly observed

Modified, from Cerletti et al., 1963

attributed to a central cholinergic block or are dependent upon other properties of the drugs. In the following section, which deals with animal investigations on atropine and related drugs, this problem will be further analyzed and discussed.

Effects of Anticholinergic Drugs on Animals

Crude observation of the symptoms of the intoxication produced by the anticholinergics in animals gives little or no indication of the type of central action of these drugs. High doses produce a syndrome of mixed excitation and depression. The hyperactivity in some animals (mice, rats), is accompanied by head swaying and exploratory behavior; in others, by a compulsive forward gait—the dog, for instance, walks into objects and attempts to "push through." The significance of these reactions is difficult to determine. Upon examination of the literature (see the review of Longo, 1966, for references relevant to the following exposition), one is impressed by the far-fetched interpretations of certain behavioral alterations described in animals. Bijlsma and Brouwer (1928) emphasize the similarities between the behavior of dogs treated with scopolamine with that of animals after decortication. Meyers and Abreu (1952) compare the syndrome due to the anticholinergics to the delirious state that occurs in the second stage of anesthesia.

It should be stressed that the effects described above are due to dosages that are many times higher than those producing the psychotomimetic syndrome in man. On the other hand, small doses do not seem to affect gross behavior at all. A better evaluation of the behavioral detriment produced by small doses is possible with more discriminating techniques and, in particular, with those related to learning and conditioning. The bulk of these experiments have been carried out with atropine and scopolamine; on the basis of these investigations, a particular profile of these two drugs emerges. These drugs proved to be very effective in disrupting reward conditioning and maze performance, however, they were relatively ineffective on conditioned avoidance. This is of interest, as it is in contrast to the effects of other central depressants (phenothiazines), which mainly block conditioned avoidance. The action of the anticholinergics most relevant to the observed effects on man is that exerted on two other aspects of learned behavior: acquisition and extinction. It has been demonstrated that these drugs exert a detrimental effect on learning processes (Figure 4.21); moreover, they provoke a "freezing" of previously learned tasks, so that these tasks become resistant to the normal extinction processes that take place in the absence of reinforcement. This interference with learning indicates an effect on the basic processes of (*a*) fixation of new experiences and (*b*) integration of the information at the level of the brain. The perseveration of response observed during the "freezing" may seem paradoxical in view of the amnesic effect of the drugs. However, extinction should be considered as capacity to learn a new task, therefore, this effect of the anticholinergic drugs can be classified as an interference with a learning process.

Another striking effect of the anticholinergics on the brain is that on cerebral electrogenesis. There seems to be no qualitative differences between the EEG alterations provoked by these drugs in the various laboratory animals. Within a short time after administration, the modifications of the tracing follow a common pattern. Bursts of 8–12 c/sec waves, similar in many aspects to the "spindles," intermingled with high-voltage slow (2–3 c/sec) waves appear in the anterior leads; slow activity is seen also in the posterior and in

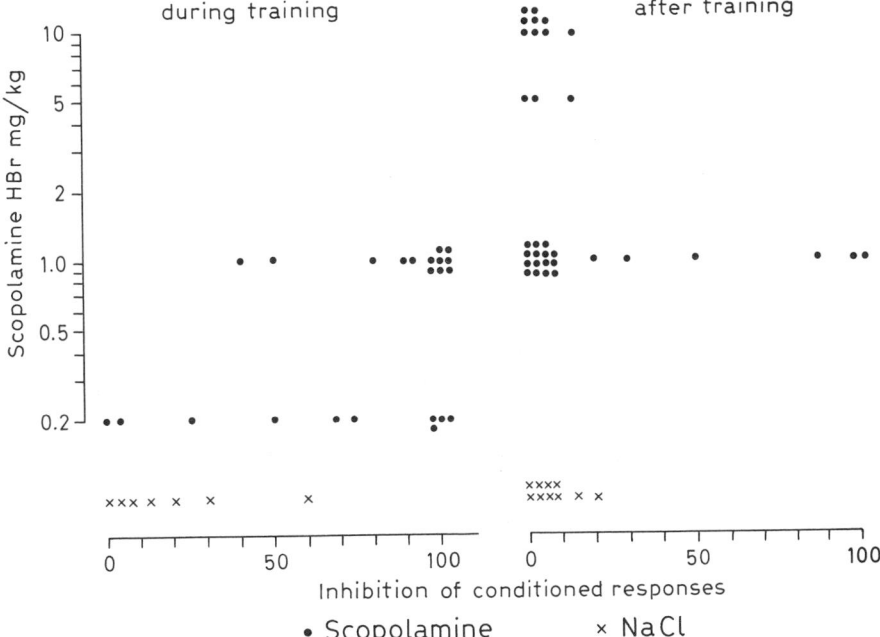

Figure 4.21
Differential effects of scopolamine on the learning and retention phase of a conditioned avoidance response in the rat. Herz studied the effects of anticholinergic drugs on the cycle of conditioning. The author used the "pole-climbing" technique and demonstrated that scopolamine, when administered during the period of formation of the avoidance reflex, caused notable alterations in the response, although it was inactive in fully trained animals (modified after Herz, 1960).

the subcortical leads. These changes are similar to those occurring during rest or sleep and are broadly classified as *EEG synchronization.* The "activating" effect of sensory stimuli on the cerebral electrical rhythms is attenuated, and with higher dosages, blocked. Also, the threshold of activation upon electrical stimulation of the reticular substance is raised. Two observations suffice to demonstrate that a central anticholinergic mechanism is involved. (1) Quaternary anticholinergics, which have a peripheral blocking potency equal or superior to that of their tertiary analogs but do not easily penetrate the cerebrum, do not synchronize the EEG. (2) The synchronization of the tracing can be reversed upon administration of cholinesterase inhibitors (eserine).

A number of anticholinergics are very active in synchronizing the EEG. Ditran, scopolamine, Ba 1443—all produce the appearance of slow waves in the EEG of the rabbit at doses below 0.1 mg/kg. Since these drugs are among the most powerful psychotomimetics, their synchronizing EEG action was related by some authors (White and Carlton, 1963) to their influence on the higher psychic processes.

Another characteristic of these drugs, first demonstrated by Wikler (1952) in the dog, is that the EEG picture of high-voltage slow activity observed after atropine is not related to the behavior of the animal; regardless of whether the animal was quiet and dozing or excited and struggling, the synchronization was always present. The relation between the EEG and behavior seen in the normal animal, in which a desynchronized EEG accompanies arousal and a synchronized EEG is observed during rest, is therefore absent (this is referred to as EEG-behavioral "dissociation"). However, the situation is not as simple as it appears from the above presentation; this problem is treated fully by several authors (see Longo, 1966). In any event, the research on animals has amply demonstrated that widespread and mutually interacting brain areas are under the control of acetylcholine and that the central anticholinergics alter in some way the normal chain of activity (Karczmar, 1969), giving rise to profound psychic and behavioral disturbances.

It should be stressed here that the hallucinogenic substances described in this chapter can be grouped in two categories, depending upon the neurochemical system upon which they impinge: (1) LSD and related substances, (2) Anticholinergics. The syndromes induced by these two types of agents suggest that two different roles are played by the two systems in question. Indeed, blockage of the acetylcholine-activated system induces a confusional state that is characterized by an estrangement from the external environment. This in turn leads to deficit of memory and learning. In contrast, the LSD-like agents, which interfere with the serotoninergic system, cause what is basically a perceptual distortion but do not induce a blockage of environmental input.

ANESTHETIC HALLUCINOGENS

It is well known that all general anesthetics may give rise to behavioral and psychic disturbances. These disturbances occur either during the phase of the loss of consciousness, which in fact is described as the state of delirium, or during the phase of recovery. This is true particularly, but not uniquely, for the volatile gaseous anesthetics. It should be remembered in this context that nitrous oxide was used as an inebriant in the 1850's, and that ether, chloroform and other volatile hydrocarbons are still used to obtain oneiroid states. A somewhat more hallucinogenic effect can be produced by such agents as phenylcyclohexylpiperidine or Sernyl.

Reviewing Sernyl, Domino (1964) appropriately describes it as a drug with a very wide spectrum of activity. This agent was shown to induce in experimental animals (particularly in the higher mammals) a state of mild sedation and tameness at small doses, and a cataleptic stupor at high doses. The investigators were impressed by the apparent depression of the sensory input, as compared to the state of the motor and neurovegetative systems, relatively unaffected; therefore, they thought of a possible application of the drug as a general anesthetic. As a matter of fact, Sernyl, administered intravenously to man in doses of 10–20 mg, proved to be a powerful agent in producing a state of unconsciousness and analgesia devoid of muscular relaxation, during which major surgical interventions could be performed. Postoperatively, however, a certain number of subjects exhibited more-or-less severe manic behavior with agitation, disorientation, vivid dreams, and hallucinations. The use of the drug in anesthetic practice was therefore curtailed, and further interest in Sernyl centered on its psychotomimetic effects and their mechanism. Experiments were carried out in normal subjects and in psychiatric patients. Diminution of sensory input was uniformly observed, together with feelings of estrangement and negativism, hypnogenic states, and repetitive motor behaviors. On the basis of these results and the fact that schizophrenic patients were especially sensitive to the drug, some authors felt that Sernyl produced, more than other drugs, the specific symptoms of schizophrenia. An hypothesis was elaborated (Luby et al., 1959) according to which the dissociative state produced by Sernyl, as well as some primary symptoms of schizophrenia, may have its basis in impaired sensory input.

Ban et al. (1961), on the other hand, were impressed by the unpleasant and frightening nature of the experience reported by the subjects treated with the drug. These authors thought that Sernyl induces the syndrome referred to in the older literature as "angor animi" or "meditatio mortis." As sensations of impending death often occur in association with vagal attacks due to bulbar lesions or irritation, the authors suggested that the medullary centers constitute the site of action of Sernyl.

References

Abood, L. G. In *Drugs Affecting the Central Nervous System*, Vol. 2, ed. by A. Burger. Marcel Dekker, New York, 1968. P. 127.

Adams, R. *Harvey Lectures* 37:168, 1942.

Adey, W. R. In *Pharmacology of Conditioning, Learning and Retention*, ed. by M. J. Mikhel'son et al. MacMillan, New York, 1964, P. 287.

Adey, W. R., et al. *Neurology* 12:591, 1962.

Aghajanian, G. K., and Bing, O. H. L. *Clin. Pharm. Ther.* 5:611, 1964.

Andén, N. E., et al. *Brit. J. Pharmacol.* 34:1, 1968.

Anichkov, S. V. In *Symposia and Special Lectures. 21st Int. Cong. Physiol. Sci.*, Buenos Aires, 1959. P. 23.

Balestrieri, A. In *Neuropsychopharmacology*, Vol. 2, ed. by E. Rothlin. Elsevier, Amsterdam, 1961. P. 44.

Ban, T. A., et al. *Can. Psychiat. Assoc. J.* 6:150, 1961.

Baran, L., et al. *J. Pharmacol.* 139:337, 1964.

Baran, L., and Longo, V. G. *Thérapie* 20:591, 1965.

Barron, F. In *LSD, Man, and Society*, ed. by R. C. De Bold and R. C. Leaf. Wesleyan, Middletown, Conn., 1967. P. 3.

Baudelaire, C. *Les Paradis Artificiels*. Poulet-Malassis, Paris, 1860.

Beccari, E. *Arch. Farm. Sper. Sci. Aff.* 61:96, 1936.

Bente, D., et al. *Arzneimittel-Forsch.* (Drug Res.) 14 (Suppl.):513, 1964.

Bijlsma, U. G., and Brouwer, J. E. *Arch. exp. Path. Pharmakol.* 138:190, 1928.

Boyd, E. S., and Meritt, D. A. *J. Pharmacol.* 149:138, 1965.

Boyd, E. S., et al. *Arch. int. Pharmacodyn.* 144:533, 1963.

Brekhman, I. I., and Sam, Y. A. In *Ethnopharmacologic Search for Psychoactive Drugs*, ed. by D. H. Efron, et al. U.S. Dept. of Health, Education and Welfare, Washington, D.C., 1967. P. 415.

Bridger, W. H., and Gantt, H. W. *Amer. J. Psychiat.* 113:352, 1956.

Brücke, F., et al. *Arch. exp. Path. Pharmakol.* 240:461, 1961.

Buck, R. W. *J. Amer. Med. Assoc.* 185:663, 1963.

Burroughs, W. *Junkie.* Olympia Press, London, 1966.

Burroughs, W., and Ginsberg, A. *The Yage Letters.* City Lights Book, New York, 1963.

Cerletti, A. In *Neuropsychopharmacology*, Vol. I, ed. by P. B. Bradley, et al. Elsevier, Amsterdam, 1959. P. 117.

Cerletti, A., et al. *Schweiz. Apoth. Ztg.* 101:210, 1963.

Chen, A. L., and Chen, K. K. *Quart. J. Pharm. Pharmacol.* 12:30, 1939.

Chorover, S. L. *J. Comp. Physiol. Psychol.* 54:649, 1961.

Cohen, S. *Psychosomatics* 7:182, 1966.

Cook, L., and Wiedley, E. *Ann. N.Y. Acad. Sci.* 66:740, 1957.

Cook, W. B., and Kieland, W. E. *J. Org. Chem.* 27:1061, 1962.

Curtis, D. R., and Davis, R. *Brit. J. Pharmacol.* 18:217, 1962.

Dagirmanjian, R., and Boyd, E. S. *J. Pharmacol.* 135:25, 1962.

Das, P. K., et al. *Arch. int. Pharmacodyn.* 135:167, 1962.

De Bold, R. C., and Leaf, R. C. *LSD, Man, and Society.* Wesleyan, Middletown, Conn., 1967. P. 212.

De Boor, W. *Pharmakopsychologie und Psychopathologie.* Springer, Berlin, 1956.

Délay, J., et al. *Presse Méd.* 81:1210, 1949.

Domino, E. F. *Int. Rev. Neurobiol.* 6:303, 1964.

Downing, D. F. *Quart. Rev.* 16:133, 1962.

Eugster, C. H. In *Ethnopharmacologic Search for Psychoactive Drugs*, ed. by D. H. Efron, et al. U.S. Dept. of Health, Education and Welfare, Washington, D.C., 1967. P. 416.

Eugster, C. H., et al. *Helv. Chim. Acta* 41:886, 1958.

Evarts, E. V. In *Chemical Concepts of Psychosis*, ed. by M. Rinkel and H. C. B. Denber. McDowell, New York, 1958. P. 41.

Fabing, H. D., and Hawkins, J. R. *Science* 123:886, 1956.

Fellows, E. J., and Cook, L. In *Psychotropic Drugs*, ed. by S. Garattini and V. Ghetti. Elsevier, Amsterdam, 1957. P. 397.

Fink, M. *EEG Clin. Neurophysiol.* 12:359, 1960.

Fink, P. J., et al. *Arch. Gen. Psychiat.* 15:209, 1966.

Florio, V., et al. *Arch. int. Pharmacodyn.* 180:81, 1969.

Flügel, F., and Bente, D. *Med. Exp.* 5:215, 1961.

Flügel, F., and Itil, T. *Psychopharmacologia* 3:79, 1962.

Forrer, G. R. *Amer. J. Psychiat.* 108:107, 1951.

Fuentes, J. A., and Longo, V. G. *Neuropharmacology* 10:15, 1971.

Fuster, J. M. *J. Nerv. Ment. Dis.* 129:252, 1959.

Gaddum, J. H. *Ann. N.Y. Acad. Sci.* 66:643, 1957.

Garriott, J. C., et al. *Life Sci.* 6:2119, 1967.

Gautier, T. Le Club des Hachichins. *La Revue des Deux Mondes*, 1 Fév. 1846.

Gayer, H. *Arch. exp. Path. Pharmakol.* 129:312, 1928.

Gershon, S., and Lang, W. J. *Arch. int. Pharmacodyn.* 135:31, 1962.

Grlič, L., and Andrec, A. *Experientia* 17:325, 1961.

Gunn, J. A. *Arch. int. Pharmacodyn.* 50:379, 1935.

Gyermek, L. *Handbook of Experimental Pharmacology* 19:507, 1966.

Haley, T. H., and Rutschmann, J. *Experientia* 13:199, 1957.

Hara, S., and Kawamori, K. *Jap. J. Pharmacol.* 3:149, 1954.

Heffter, A. *Arch. exp. Path. Pharmakol.* 4:418, 1897.

Heim, R., and Wasson, R. G. *Les Champignons Halluciogènes du Mexique*. Editions du Muséum National d'Historie Naturelle, Paris, 1958.

Herz, A. *Z. Biol.* 112:104, 1960.

Hess, G., and Jacobsen, E. *Acta Pharm. Tox.* 13:125, 1957.

Himwich, H. E., et al. In *Neuropsychopharmacology*, ed. by P. B. Bradley, et al. Elsevier, Amsterdam, 1959, P. 329.

Himwich, W. A., et al. In *Recent Advances in Biol. Psychiat.*, ed. by J. Wortis. Grune and Stratton, New York, 1960. P. 321.

Hochstein, F. A. and Paradies, A. M. *J. Am. Chem. Soc.* 79:5735, 1957.

Hoffer, A., and Osmond, H. *The Hallucinogens*. Academic Press, New York, 1967.

Hofmann, A. In *Drugs Affecting the Central Nervous System*, Vol. 2, ed. by A. Burger. Dekker, New York, 1968. P. 169.

Hofmann, A., and Cerletti, A. *Deut. Med. Wochschr.* 86:885, 1961.

Hofmann, A., and Tscherter, A. *Experientia* 16:414, 1960.

Hollister, L. E., and Friedhoff, A. J. *Nature* 210:1377, 1966.

Holmstedt, B. *Arch. int. Pharmacodyn.* 156:285, 1965.

Isbell, H. *Psychopharmacologia* 1:29, 1959.

Isbell, H. In *Ethnopharmacologic Search for Psychoactive Drugs*, ed. by D. H. Efron, et al. U.S. Dept. of Health, Education and Welfare, Washington, D.C., 1967. P. 377.

Isbell, H., and Gorodetski, C. W. *Psychopharmacologia* 8:331, 1966.

Isbell, H., et al. *Psychopharmacologia* 1:20, 1959.

Isbell, H., et al. *Psychopharmacologia* 2:147, 1961.

Isbell, H., et al. In *Neuropsychopharmacology*, ed. by P. B. Bradley, et al. Elsevier, Amsterdam, 1964. P. 440.

Isbell, H., et al. *Psychopharmacologia* 2:184, 1967.

Itil, T., and Fink, M. In *Anticholinergic Drugs*, ed. by P. B. Bradley and M. Fink. Elsevier, Amsterdam, 1968. P. 149.

Jacobsen, E. *Clin. Pharmacol.* 4:480, 1963.

Jarvik, M. E., and Chorover, S. *Psychopharmacologia* 1:221, 1960.

Kabelik, J., et al. *Bulletin on Narcotics* 12:5, 1960.

Kant, F., and Krapf, E. *Arch. exp. Path. Pharmakol.* 129:319, 1928.

Karczmar, A. G. *Actualités Pharmacol.* 22:293, 1969.

Key, B. J. *Brit. Med. Bull.* 21:30, 1965.

Kinross-Wright, V. J. In *Neuropsychopharmacology*, Vol. I, ed. by P. B. Bradley, et al. Elsevier, Amsterdam, 1959. P. 453.

Klüver, H. *Mescal: the Divine Plant.* Kegan, London, 1928.

Kögl, F., et al. *Rec. Trav. Chim.* 76:109, 1957.

Korte, F., and Sieper, H. In *Hashish: Its Chemistry and Pharmacology* (Ciba Found. Study Group N. 21). Churchill, London, 1965. P. 15.

Lambert, P. A., et al. In *Neuropsychopharmacology*, Vol. 3, ed. by E. Rothlin. Elsevier, Amsterdam, 1961. P. 374.

Lewin, L. *The Therapeutic Gazette* 4:231, 1888.

Lewin, L. *Phantastica. Die Betäubenden und Erregenden Genussmittel.* Georg Stilke, Berlin, 1924.

Liataud, A. *Compt. Rend. Acad. Sci.* 18:146, 1844.

Lipparini, F., et al. *Physiol. Behav.* 4:527, 1969.

Loewe, S. *Arch. exp. Path. Pharmakol.* 211:175, 1950.

Longo, V. G. *Pharmacol. Rev.* 18:965, 1966.

Luby, E. D., et al. *Arch. Neurol. Psychiat.* 81:363, 1959.

Mantegazzini, P. *Handbuch exper. Pharmacol.* 19:424, 1966.

McGaugh, J. L., et al. *Psychopharmacologia* 4:126, 1963.

McIsaac, W. M. *Biochim. Biophys. Acta* 52:607, 1961.

Marinesco, G. *Presse Médicale* 74:1433, 1933.

Meyers, F. H., and Abreu, B. F. *J. Pharmacol.* 104:387, 1952.

Miller, J. J. *J. Nerv. Ment. Dis.* 124:260, 1956.

Monnier, M., and Krupp, P. *Arch. int. Pharmacodyn.* 127:337, 1960.

Naranjo, C. In *Ethnopharmacologic Search for Psychoactive Drugs*, ed. by D. H. Efron, et al. U.S. Dept. of Health, Education and Welfare, Washington, D.C., 1967. P. 385.

Osmond, H. *J. Mental Sci.* 101:526, 1955.

Osmond, H. *Ann. N.Y. Acad. Sci.* 66:418, 1957.

Osmond, H., and Smythies, J. *J. Mental Sci.* 98:309, 1952.

Ostfeld, A. M., and Aruguete, A. *J. Pharmacol.* 137:133, 1962.

Panorama Sandoz, March-April 1968.

Pennes, H. H., and Hoch, P. H. *Amer. J. Psychiat.* 113:887, 1957.

Pfeiffer, C. C. *Int. Rev. Neurobiol.* 1:195, 1959.

Poirier, L. J., et al. *Can. J. Physiol. Pharmacol.* 46:585, 1968.

Poisson, J. *Ann. Pharm. Franc.* 23:241, 1965.

Purpura, D. *Arch. Neurol. Psychiat.* 75:132, 1956.

Ray, O. S., and Marrazzi, A. S. *Science* 133:1705, 1961.

Reti, L. In *The Alkaloids*, Vol. III, ed. by R. H. F. Manske and H. L. Holmes. Academic Press, New York, 1953. P. 313.

Reti, L. In *The Alkaloids*, Vol. IV, ed. by R. H. F. Manske and H. L. Holmes. Academic Press, New York, 1954. P. 7.

Rinaldi, F. *J. Nerv. Ment. Dis.* 126:272, 1958.

Rinkel, M., et al. In *Neuropsychopharmacology*, ed. by E. Rothlin. Elsevier, Amsterdam, 1961, P. 273.

Roth, W. T. *Psychopharmacologia* 9:253, 1966.

Rothlin, E. *J. Pharm. Pharmacol.* 9:569, 1957.

Rouhier, A. *Le Peyote. C. Doin*, Paris, 1927.

Sadowski, B., and Longo, V. G. *EEG Clin. Neurophysiol.* 14:465, 1962.

Schallek, W. and Smith, T. H. F. *J. Pharmacol.* 104:291, 1952.

Schultes, R. E. *A Contribution to our Knowledge of Rivea corymbosa, the Narcotic ololiuqui of the Aztecs.* Botanical Museum of Harvard University, Cambridge, Mass., 1941.

Schweigerdt, A. K., et al. *J. Pharmacol.* 151:353, 1966.

Seitz, G. In *Ethnopharmacologic Search for Psychoactive Drugs*, ed. by D. H. Efron, et al. U.S. Dept. of Health, Education and Welfare, Washington, D.C., 1967. P. 315.

Shore, P. A., et al. *Science* 122:284, 1955.

Shulgin, A. T. *Experientia* 20:366, 1964.

Shulgin, A. T. *Nature* 210:380, 1966.

Shulgin, A. T., et al. *Nature* 189:1011, 1961.

Shulgin, A. T., et al. *Nature* 221:537, 1969.

Sigg, E. B., et al. *Arch. int. Pharmacodyn.* 149:164, 1964.

Sivadjian, J. *Compt. Rend. Acad. Sci.* 199:884, 1934.

Smythies, J. R., et al. *Psychopharmacologia* 10:379, 1967a.

Smythies, J. R., et al. *Nature* 216:128, 1967b.

Snyder, S. H., et al. *Science* 158:669, 1967.

Solms, H. *J. Clin. Exp. Psychopath.* 17:429, 1956.

Speck, L. B. *J. Pharmacol.* 119:78, 1957.

Speck, L. B. *J. Pharmacol.* 122:201, 1958.

Stoll, W. A. *Schweiz. Arch. Neurol. Psychiat.* 60:279, 1947.

Stoll, A., et al. *Experientia* 11:396, 1955.

Sturtevant, F. M., and Drill, V. A. *Proc. Soc. Exper. Biol. Med.* 92:383, 1956.

Szara, S. In *Psychotropic Drugs*, ed. by S. Garattini and V. Ghetti. Elsevier, Amsterdam, 1957. P. 460.

Taylor, D. In *Ethnopharmacologic Search for Psychoactive Drugs*, ed. by D. H. Efron, et al. U.S. Dept. of Health, Education and Welfare, Washington, D.C., 1967. P. 392.

Theobald W., et al. *Arzneimittel-Forsch.* (Drug Res.) 18:311, 1968.

Turner, W. J., and Merlis, S. *Arch. Neurol. Psychiat.* 81:121, 1959.

Vojtechovsky, M., et al. In *Anticholinergic Drugs*, ed. by P. B. Bradley and M. Fink. Elsevier, Amsterdam, 1968. P. 86.

Waser, P. In *Ethnopharmacologic Search for Psychoactive Drugs*, ed. by D. H. Efron, et al. U.S. Dept. of Health, Education and Welfare, Washington, D.C., 1967. P. 419.

Wasson, R. G. In *Ethnopharmacologic Search for Psychoactive Drugs*, ed. by D. H. Efron, et al. U.S. Dept. of Health, Education and Welfare, Washington, D.C., 1967. P. 405.

West, L. J., et al. *Science* 138:1100, 1962.

White, R. P., and Carlton, R. A. *Psychopharmacologia* 4:459, 1963.

Wikler, A. *Proc. Soc. Exp. Biol.* 79:261, 1952.

Woolley, D. W. *The Biochemical Bases of Psychoses*, Wiley, New York, 1962.

Zetler, G. *Arch. exp. Path. Pharmakol.* 231:34, 1957.

Glossary-Index

This Glossary-Index briefly defines technical terms that are not defined in the text. It also lists the numbers of pages on which particular drugs and other subjects are mentioned or discussed. Words set in SMALL CAPS in the definitions are listed elsewhere in the Glossary-Index.

ABERRANT. Wandering from a normal course.

ABREACTION. Release of emotional tension by recreating a disagreeable experience in words, actions or imaginings.

ACETYLCHOLINE. Chemical mediator of the CHOLINERGIC system at the central and peripheral nervous system.

ACETYLCHOLINESTERASE. Enzyme that hydrolizes ACETYLCHOLINE and other CHOLINE esters.

ACROAGONINE. Putative substance liberated in the brain by ELECTRO-SHOCK treatment.

ADJUNCTIVE. Assisting or aiding.

ADJUVANT. A drug used in conjunction with another drug to aid its action.

ADRENERGIC. Activated or transmitted by EPINEPHRINE; a term applied to sympathetic nerve fibers.

ADRENOGLOMERULOTROPINE. Hormone secreted by the epiphysis (*see* page 138).

ADRENOLYTIC. Inhibiting the action of ADRENERGIC nerves; inhibiting the response to EPINEPHRINE.

ADRENOMIMETIC. Mimicking the action of EPINEPHRINE.

AFFECTIVE. Pertaining to feelings or emotions.

AJMALINE. An ALKALOID extracted from Rauwolfia (*see* RAUWOLFIA SERPENTINA).

AKATHISIA. Restlessness.

ALIPHATIC. This term is applied to hydrocarbons in which the carbon atoms are linked in open chains rather than in closed rings.

ALKALOID. A large group of physiologically active nitrogen-containing organic bases found in plants. (Examples are ATROPINE, caffeine, COCAINE, morphine, nicotine, quinine, strychnine.)

AMANITA. Species of poisonous mushrooms, as the fly agaric (*see* page 143).

AMBIENT. Surrounding; milieu.

AMITRIPTYLINE. Drug used in the treatment of DEPRESSIONS (*see* page 51).

AMNESIA. Lack or loss of memory.

AMPHETAMINE. Central nervous system stimulant, belonging to the class of ADRENERGIC drugs.

AMYGDALA. Rounded mass lying deep within the ventrolateral part of the brain.

ANALOG. A compound with a structure similar to that of another compound, but differing in some detail.

ANALONIUM WILLIAMSI. The cactus peyotl (*see* PEYOTE).

ANESTHESIA. Loss of sensation.

ANGOR ANIMI. Latin term for a feeling of impending doom.

ANHALONIDINE. An ALKALOID found in PEYOTE (*see* page 102).

ANHALONINE. An ALKALOID found in PEYOTE (*see* page 102).

ANTIEMETIC. Curing or preventing nausea and vomiting.

ANTIHISTAMINIC. Counteracting the effects of histamine.

ANTI-INFLAMMATORY. Counteracting or suppressing inflammation.

ANTIMONOAMINEOXIDASE. Blocking the effects of the enzyme monoamine oxidase (MAO; *see* page 59).

ANTIPARKINSONIAN. Drug used for the treatment of PARKINSONISM.

ANTIPSYCHOTIC. Curing mental aberrations.

ANTIPUTREFACTIVE. Counteracting putrefaction of food.

ANTIPYRETIC. Reducing fever.

ANTISEROTONINIC. Counteracting the effects of SEROTONIN.

ANTITUSSIVE. A drug that relieves coughing.

ANXIETY. Fearful anticipation of unpleasant events, often accompanied by feelings of isolation and helplessness.

ANXIOLYTIC. A drug that cures ANXIETY.

APOCYNACEAE. Family of plants.

APOMORPHINE. An ALKALOID derived from morphine; induces EMESIS.

ARECOLINE. An ALKALOID contained in the nut of a genus of palm trees, chiefly Asiatic.

AREFLEXIA. Absence of reflexes.

ARMAMENTARIUM. Complete resources of a medical specialist, including books, drugs, instruments, and so forth.

ASARONE. *See* page 112.

ATARAXIA. Calmness or peacefulness.

ATHETOSIS. Continual slow movements, especially of the extremities; often due to brain damage.

ATROPA BELLADONNA. Genus of SOLANACEAE, rich in ALKALOIDS of the ATROPINE group (*see* page 155).

ATROPINE. An ALKALOID found in several species of plants (*see* page 155).

AUTONOMIC SYSTEM. That part of the nervous system that functions independently of the will. Also called NEUROVEGETATIVE SYSTEM.

AXODENDRITIC SYNAPSE. Junction between axon terminals and dendrites of a neuron.

BACTERIOSTATIC. Inhibiting the growth or multiplication of bacteria.

BANISTERIOPSIS CAAPI (MALPIGHIACEAE). Genus of tropical plants used in the preparation of HALLUCINOGENIC concoctions (*see* page 136).

BANISTERIOPSIS RUSBYANA. *See above.*

BARBITURATE. A salt of barbituric acid; any of a group of barbituric acid derivatives used as sedatives, hypnotics or anticonvulsants.

BENACTYZINE. *See* pages 2, 157, 158.

BENPERIDOL. *See* page 37.

BENZAZOLE. *See* page 84.

BENZEDRINE. Registered trade mark for a brand of AMPHETAMINE.

BENZODIAZEPINE. *See* page 87.

BENZOQUINOLINE. *See* page 33.

3, 1, 4-BENZOXADIAZEPINE. *See* page 87.

BETTA SPLENDENS. Aquarium fighting fish used for psychopharmacological assays.

BLOCKADE. Block or inhibition of an effect.

BRADYCARDIA. Abnormally slow heartbeat.

BRAINSTEM. That part of the brain consisting of the medulla oblongata, pons, and MESENCEPHALON.

BROM-SUBSTITUTED LSD. *See* pages 119, 122.

BUFOTENINE. *See* page 132.

BULBOCAPNINE. Alkaloid isolated from the plant *Corydalis cava*, which, injected into animals, induces a state of CATALEPSY.

BUTYROPHENONE. *See* page 35.

CANNABIDIOL. *See* page 151.

CANNABIDIOLIC ACID. *See* page 151.

CANNABIGEROL. *See* page 151.

CANNABINOL. *See* page 151.

CANNABIS INDICA. *See* page 147.

CANNABIS SATIVA. *See* page 147.

CARAMIPHEN. *See* pages 2, 157.

β-CARBOLINE. *See* page 136.

CARCINOID. A yellow circumscribed tumor found in the stomach or intestine.

CARISOPRODOL. *See* page 76.

CAROTID. Artery of the neck, supplying blood to the brain.

CARPOPHORE. The umbrella-like top of a mushroom.

CATABOLITE. Any product of a destructive metabolic process.

CATALEPSY. Condition characterized by waxy rigidity.

CATALEPTIGENIC. A substance that induces a state of CATALEPSY.

CATATONIA. Often used as a synonym for CATALEPSY.

CATECHOLAMINES. Derivatives of catechol, containing an amino group; EPINEPHRINE, NOREPINEPHRINE, and DOPAMINE are catecholamines and play the role of chemical mediators in organisms.

CAUDAL. Pertaining to the posterior parts of the brain; opposite of ROSTRAL.

CEREBROSPINAL AXIS. The entire central nervous system, from brain through spinal cord.

CHEMOTHERAPY. The treatment of disease by administering chemicals.

CHOLINERGIC. Stimulated, activated or transmitted by ACETYLCHOLINE.

CHLORAL HYDRATE. General anesthetic (*see* page 89).

CHLORDIAZEPOXIDE. *See* page 88.

p-CHLOROMETAMPHETAMINE. *See* page 33.

p-CHLOROPHENYLALANINE. *See* pages 33, 35.

CHLORPROMAZINE (CPZ). *See* page 8.

CHOLINE. Quaternary base present in many animal tissues.

CHOLINESTERASE. *See* ACETYLCHOLINESTERASE.

CHOREIFORM MOVEMENT. Involuntary and irregular jerking movement.

CICATRICIAL LESION. Alteration produced by a scar.

CLAVICEPS PURPUREA. Genus of fungi that infests various plants (*see* page 113).

CLONIC MOVEMENT. Jerking, more or less intense.

COAXIHUITL. *See* page 141.

COCAINE. An ALKALOID extracted from the leaves of coca, possessing local anesthetic and central-nervous-system excitatory properties.

COCKTAIL LYTIQUE. A French term for a mixture of drugs used to block the functions of the AUTONOMIC and central nervous system, thus producing the state known as artificial hibernation.

CONJUNCTIVAL SAC. The space between the eyeball and the lower eyelid.

CONVOLVULACEAE. Family of twining plants that includes the morning glory (*see* page 141).

CONVULSION. Violent involuntary contraction of the skeletal muscles; it can be persistent (tonic) or alternating with relaxation (clonic).

COPROLALIA. Utterance of filthy words.

CPZ (CHLORPROMAZINE). *See* page 8.

CURAROMIMETIC. Mimicking the effect of curare (paralysis of voluntary muscles).

CYCLOHEPTADIENE. Compound containing a conjugated seven-membered ring. *See* page 51.

DATURA METELOIDES. Genus of plants of the ATROPINE group; rich in ALKALOIDS.

DATURA STRAMONIUM. Genus of plants of the ATROPINE group; rich in ALKALOIDS.

DECOCTION. Medicine or other substance prepared by boiling.

DELIRIUM TREMENS. A Latin term for acute mental disturbance, usually characterized by motor excitement and mental confusion.

DEPRESSANT. A substance that produces DEPRESSION.

DEPRESSION. *See* page 47.

DEPRESSIVE. Pertaining to DEPRESSION.

DESERPIDINE. *See* page 28.

DESIPRAMINE. *See* page 52.

DEXTROMORAMIDE. *See* page 38.

DIAZEPAM (VALIUM). *See* page 88.

DIENCEPHALON. Part of the brain, including the thalamus and hypothalamus.

DIETHAZINE. *See* page 25.

DIETHYLPROPANEDIOL. *See* page 84.

DIETHYLTRYPTAMINE. *See* page 135.

DIHYDROHARMINE. Or harmaline (*see* page 139).

1,2-DIMETHYLHEPTYLPYRANE (DMHP). *See* page 152.

DIMETHYLTRYPTAMINE. *See* page 135.

DIPHENHYDRAMINE. An ANHIHISTAMINIC drug (*see* page 2).

DIPHENYLHYDANTOIN. Drug used in the therapy of epilepsy (*see* pages 87, 93).

DISEQUILIBRIUM. Unstable condition, either physical or mental.

DITRAN. *See* page 158.

DOPA. Dihydroxyphenylalanine, a precursor of DOPAMINE and NOREPINEPHRINE (*see* page 41).

DOPAMINE. A CATECHOLAMINE, present in the brain, where it plays a role as a chemical mediator.

DOPAMINERGIC. Pertaining to or acting like DOPAMINE.

DROPERIDOL. *See* pages 37, 38.

DUBOISIA MYOPOROIDES. Plant containing ATROPINE or related ALKALOIDS.

DYSFUNCTION. Alteration of normal function.

DYSPHORIA. Altered mental state, combining elation and DEPRESSION.

DYSTONIA-DYSKINESIA. Alteration in voluntary movements.

DYSURIA. Alteration in urination.

ECHOLALIA. Meaningless repetition by a patient of words addressed to him.

ELECTROPHORESIS. Migration of particles under the influence of an electric field.

ELECTROSHOCK. Shock (usually motor CONVULSIONS) produced by application of electric current to the brain.

ELEMICIN. *See* page 109.

EMATURIA. Presence of blood in the urine.

EMESIS. Vomiting.

ENDOGENOUS. Originating within the organism.

ENURESIS. Involuntary discharge of urine.

EPINEPHRINE. Adrenal hormone that stimulates autonomic nerve action. *See* pages 59, 60.

ERGOTAMINE. ALKALOID present in the CLAVICEPS PURPUREA; it has ADRENOLYTIC properties.

ESERINE. An ALKALOID found in the Calabar bean; it has anticholinesterasic activity. Also called PHYSOSTIGMINE (*see* pages 35, 157).

EXTRAPYRAMIDAL. Central motor mechanisms that are not mediated through the pyramidal tract.

FENTANYL. *See* page 38.

FLUANISONE. *See* pages 37, 38.

GAMMA MOTONEURONAL LOOP. Neural loop that regulates muscle tonus; comprising afferent proprioceptive input and and efferent motor system.

GANGLIONIC. Pertaining to the ganglia (relay stations) of the AUTONOMIC SYSTEM.

GANGLIOPLEGIC PROPERTY. Ability to block nervous transmission at the level of the ganglia.

GENICULATE BODY. Part of the brain; the visual pathways from the eye to the cortex pass through the lateral geniculate body, which is located in the MESENCEPHALON.

GILLES DE LA TOURETTE'S DISEASE. *See* page 37.

GLUCOSIDE. Natural product containing a carbohydrate (usually sugar) molecule.

GLYCEROL ETHERS. *See* page 74.

GYNECOMASTIA. Excessive development of the mammary glands in the male, even including the production of milk.

HALLUCINATION. Sense perception not founded upon objective reality.

HALLUCINOGENIC. A drug or treatment that induces HALLUCINATIONS or distortions in the perception of reality.

HALOPERDOL. *See* page 37.

HARMANE. *See* page 139.

HARMINE. *See* page 136.

HARMOL. *See* page 139.

HEMIBALLISMUS. Motor restlessness involving half of the body.

HEMINEURINE. Vitamin B_1 (*see* page 38).

HEPATO-TOXIC. Toxic to the liver.

HETEROCYCLIC. A chemical having a closed molecular ring that includes atoms of different elements.

HIPPOCAMPUS. Curved structure on the floor of the lateral ventricle, also called Ammon's horn.

HOMOLATERAL. Of the same side.

HOMOVANILLIC ACID. A product of metabolism of the CATECHOLAMINES.

HORRIPILATION. Piloerection in animals; goose flesh in man.

5-HYDROXYDIMETHYLTRYPTAMINE. Bufotenine (*see* page 132).

HYDROXYDIONE. *See* page 38.

5-HYDROXYINDOLACETIC ACID. A CATABOLITE of SEROTONIN (*see* page 60).

5-HYDROXYTRYPTOPHAN. A precursor of SEROTONIN.

HYOSCYAMINE. *See* page 155.

HYOSCYAMUS NIGER. Plant containing SCOPOLAMINE (*see* page 155).

HYPERGLYCEMIA. Concentration of glucose in the blood above the normal limits.

HYPERIRRITABILITY. Abnormal responsiveness to slight stimuli.

HYPERPNEA. Increase of the depth and rate of respiration.

HYPERPYREXIA. Fever.

HYPERREACTIVITY. *See* HYPERIRRITABILITY.

HYPERREFLEXIA. Exaggeration of reflexes.

HYPERSEROTONINEMIA. High content of SEROTONIN in the blood.

HYPERTENSIVE PATIENT. Patient with high blood pressure.

HYPERTONIA. Excessive tone, or tension, of the muscles.

HYPNOGENIC. Inducing sleep.

HYPOGEOUS TUBERCLE. Small round mass of plant tissue beneath the surface of the ground, usually growing from the roots of a plant.

HYPOMANIA. A mild mania.

HYPOTENSION. Low blood pressure.

HYPOTONIA. Low tone, or tension, of the muscles.

IBOTENIC ACID. *See* page 146.

IMIPRAMINE. *See* page 50.

INCOORDINATION. Lack of coordination of movements.

INDOLAMINE. Chemical containing an INDOLE ring and an amino group (NH_2); SEROTONIN is an example.

INDOLE. A five-element chemical ring, containing a nitrogen atom.

INSUFFLATE. To blow into.

INTERNEURON. An internuncial, or linking, neuron.

INTRACAROTID INJECTION. Administration of a drug into the CAROTID artery.

IPOMOEA VIOLACEA. *See* page 141.

IPRONIAZID. *See* page 59.

ISONIAZID. *See* page 50.

ISOQUINOLINE. *See* page 101.

LA 111. *See* page 142.

LACRIMAL. Pertaining to the tear-producing glands.

LARGACTIL. *Registered trade mark* for CHLORPROMAZINE *(see* page 26).

LATAH. *See* page 37.

L-DOPA. *See* DOPA.

LEGUMINOSAE. Family of plants characterized by fruits that are legumes.

LEVOROTATORY. A compound that (because of the structural characteristics of its molecule) rotates the plane of polarized light to the left when in solution.

LOPHOPHORA WILLIAMSI. *See* page 100.

LOPHOPHORINE. *See* page 102.

LSD. *See* page 113.

LYTIC EFFECT. Dissolution; remission (a lessening of intensity).

MACROPSIA. Seeing objects as larger than they are in reality.

MAO (MONOAMINE OXIDASE). Enzyme that inactivates the biological MONOAMINES by oxidation.

MARIHUANA. Or marijuana *(see* page 147).

MEBUTAMATE. *See* page 76.

MECHANISM OF ACTION. The process underlying or responsible for a natural phenomenon.

MEDITATIO MORTIS. Feeling of oncoming death.

MENTATION. Mental functioning.

MEPAZINE. *See* page 9.

MEPERIDINE. *See* page 35.

MEPHENESIN. *See* page 74.

MEPROBAMATE. *See* page 74.

MESCAL. *See* PEYOTE.

MESCALINE. *See* page 99.

MESENCEPHALON. Or midbrain. One of the sections in which the brain is divided.

METABOLITE. Any product of a metabolic process (*see also* CATAB-OLITE).

METHAMINODIAZEPOXIDE. *See* page 87.

p-METHOXYAMPHETAMINE. *See* page 108.

5-METHOXYDIMETHYLTRYPTAMINE. *See* page 133.

6-METHOXYHARMALAN. *See* page 138.

3-METHOXY-4-HYDROXYMANDELIC ACID. *See* page 63.

2-5-METHOXY-4-METHYLAMPHETAMINE. *See* page 109.

METHOXYMETHYLENDIOXYAMPHETAMINE. *See* page 108.

METHOXYPHENYLETHYLAMINE. *See* page 107.

METHOXYPHENYLISOPROPYLAMINE. *See* page 107.

1, 2, 4-TRIMETHOXY-5-PROPENYLBENZENE. *See* page 113.

6-METHOXYTETRAHYDROHARMAN. *See* page 138.

α-METHYL DOPA. *See* page 33.

α-METHYLPARATYROSINE. *See* page 33.

2-METHYL-2-N-PROPYL-1-2-PROPANEDIOL DICARBAMATE. *See* page 74.

3-METHYLHARMANE. *See* page 140.

METHYLPERIDOL (MOPERONE). *See* page 37.

METHYSERGIDE. *See* page 70.

MEZCALINE. Or mescaline. *See* page 99.

MG/KG. Milligram per kilogram of body weight. When administered to laboratory animals, the dosage of a drug is usually referred to body weight. This procedure is rarely applied to man.

MICROSOMAL. Pertaining to microsomes (cell particles); microsomes are one of the subcellular elements of protoplasm.

MIDCOLLICULAR PREPONTINE TRANSECTION. Type of surgical intervention, disconnecting the ROSTRAL part of the brain from the CAUDAL part at a specified location.

MIDPONTINE PRETRIGEMINAL. *See preceding term.* The same type of surgical intervention, except at a different specified location.

MIOSIS. Constriction of the pupil.

MONOAMINE. Compound containing an amino group (NH_2).

MONOAMINE OXIDASE. *See* MAO.

MONOSYNAPTIC. A neuronal circuit that includes only one synapse.

MOTONEURONE. A neurone that innervates voluntary muscles.

MOTOR DEPRESSION. Impairment of voluntary motility.

MUSCARINE. *See* page 145.

MUSCAZONE. *See* page 145.

MYDRIASIS. Dialation of the pupil.

MYOCARDIAL. Pertaining to the heart muscle.

MYOCLONUS. Clonic spasm of a muscle or of a group of muscles.

MYORELAXANT. A drug that induces a relaxation of muscle tension.

MYRISTICA FRAGRANS. Nutmeg (*see* page 112).

MYRISTICIN. *See* page 112.

NEUROLEPTIC. A drug depressing the central nervous system.

NEUROPHARMACOLOGY. Branch of pharmacology that studies the effects of drugs on the central nervous system.

NEUROPSYCHOPHARMACOLOGY. *See* NEUROPHARMACOLOGY.

NEUROVEGETATIVE. *See* AUTONOMIC.

NICTITATING MEMBRANE. The third eyelid, hinged at the inner side of the lower lid of the eye of various animals.

NIGRO-STRIATAL. System formed by the substantia nigra and the corpora striata, part of the EXTRAPYRAMIDAL pathway.

NITRAZEPAM. *See* page 89.

NOREPINEPHRINE. *See* CATECHOLAMINES.

NORHARMANE. *See* page 139.

OCULOGYRIC CRISIS. Movements of the eye about the anteroposterior axis.

OLOLIUQUI. *See* page 141.

ONIROID. Dreamlike.

OPISTHOTONOS. Tetanic spasm of the muscles in which the head and the heels are bent backward.

ORTHOGRAPHY. Correct spelling and writing.

ORTHOPEDICS. Branch of medicine dealing with the treatment of deformities, diseases, and injuries of the bone and joints.

ORTHOSTATIC. Pertaining to or caused by standing erect.

ORTHOTOLUOLOXYPROPANEDIOL. *See* MEPHENESIN.

OXAZEPAM. *See* page 92.

PALPEBRAL PTOSIS. Drooping of the upper eyelid.

PANTHERINE. *See* page 145.

PARANOIA. A mental disorder characterized by ambitions or suspicions.

PARENTERALLY. Administration of a drug not through the alimentary canal.

PARESTHESIA. Morbid or abnormal sensation.

PARGYLINE. *See* page 62.

PARKINSONISM. Chronic condition marked by rigidity and tremor.

PATELLAR REFLEX. Kneejerk.

PEGANUM HARMALA. *See* page 136

PENTAMETHYLENTETRAZOL. Synthetic compound with convulsant properties (*see* pages 68, 91).

PENTOBARBITAL. General anesthetic, belonging to the BARBITURATE group.

PEYOTE. *See* page 99.

PHENAGLYCODOL. *See* page 76.

PHENIPRAZIN. *See* page 62.

PHENOBARBITAL. Anticonvulsant drug belonging to the BARBITU-RATE group (*see* page 89).

PHENOTHIAZINE. *See* page 7.

PHENYLCYCLOHEXYLPIPERIDINE. *See* page 163.

PHENYLETHYLAMINE. *See* page 108.

PHENYRAMIDOL. *See page* 76.

PILZATROPINE. *See* page 145.

PIPERIDYL BENZYLATES. *See* page 158.

PIPTADENIA. *See* page 132.

PNEUMOENCEPHALOGRAPHY. X-ray examination of the brain after injection of air into the cerebral ventricles.

POLYURIA. Increased excretion of urine.

POSTENCEPHALITIC. Occurring after or in consequence of an encephalitis (inflammation of the brain).

POSTTRAUMATIC. Occurring after or in consequence of an injury.

POTENTIATE. Enhance.

PRENYLAMINE (SEGONTIN). *See* page 33.

PRINCIPLE, ACTIVE. The constituent in a mixture of compounds that is responsible for a pharmacological action.

PROCAINE. Synthetic compound possessing local anesthetic properties.

PROCHLORPERAZINE. *See* page 25.

PROMETHAZINE. *See* page 2.

PROPANOLOL. *See* page 70.

PROPRIOCEPTOR. Sensory nerve terminal that gives information on movements and position of the body.

PSEUDORESERPINE. *See* page 29.

PSILOCYBE MEXICANA. *See* page 128.

PSILOCYBE SEMPERVIVA, P. WASSONII, P. AZTECORUM, P. YUNGENSIS. *See* page 130.

PSILOCYBIN. *See* page 127.

PSYCHEDELIC. *See* page 98.

PSYCHODYSLEPTIC. A drug that induces alterations in mental functioning.

PSYCHOMOTOR AGITATION. Increase of psychic and motor activity.

PSYCHOTIC SYNDROME. Severe mental disorder, such as SCHIZO-PHRENIA.

PSYCHOTOGENIC. A drug or treatment that induces a psychotic state.

PSYCHOTROPIC. A drug that affects the psyche.

RAUNESCINE. *See* page 29.

RAUWOLFIA SERPENTINA. *See* page 27.

RECRUITING RESPONSE. *See* page 85.

RESCINAMINE. *See* page 28.

RESERPINE. *See* page 27.

RETICULAR FORMATION. *See* pages 24, 84, 86.

RETICULOCORTICAL. Nervous pathways between the RETICULAR FORMATION and the cerebral cortex and vice versa.

RHINENCEPHALON. Portion of the brain, including the HIPPOCAM-PUS, AMYGDALA, and the limbic cortex.

RIVEA CORYMBOSA. *See* page 141.

RO 4-1254. *See* page 69.

ROSTRAL. Pertaining to the anterior parts of the brain; opposite of CAUDAL.

RP 4560. *See* page 8.

SCHIZOPHRENIA. A PSYCHOTIC SYNDROME characterized by serious alteration of the mental processes.

SCOPOLAMINE. *See* page 155.

SCOPOLIA JAPONICA. Plant containing SCOLOPAMINE (*see* page 155).

SERNYL. *See* page 163.

SEROTONIN. Also called 5-hydoxytryptamine; thought to act at synapses as a chemical mediator. *See* INDOLAMINE.

SEROTONINERGIC. Pertaining to or acting like SEROTONIN.

SERPENTINE. *See* page 28.

SERPENTININE. *See* page 28.

SHOCK THERAPY. Treatment of psychotic patients by induction of coma or CONVULSIONS, using drugs or by passing electric current through the brain.

SLOW-WAVE SLEEP. State of sleep accompanied by the presence of slow, large-amplitude waves in the EEG.

SOLANACEAE. Family of plants rich in ATROPINE and SCOPOLAMINE.

SPASMOLYTIC. An agent that relieves spasm.

SPECTROFLUORIMETRIC. A method for estimating a substance in a liquid, as indicated by its spectrum and its fluorescence.

SPINAL ANIMAL. Animal in which the connection between the spinal cord and the brain is surgically severed.

SPIROPERIDOL. *See* page 41.

STEREOTAXY. Approach to the internal nuclei of the brain by means of external coordinates.

STEREOTYPIC. Persistant repetition of senseless acts or words.

STP. *See* page 109.

STRIATUM. Part of the brain, made up of the caudate nucleus, putamen, and the lentiform nucleus.

STROPHARIA. *See* page 128.

STRYCHNINE. Convulsant drug (*see* page 128).

SUPRASPINAL. Above the spinal cord.

SYMPATHERGIC. *See* SYMPATHOMIMETIC.

SYMPATHOLYTIC. *See* ADRENOLYTIC.

SYMPATHOMIMETIC. *See* ADRENOMIMETIC.

SYNDROME. A set of symptoms that occur together.

TACHYCARDIA. Abnormally fast heartbeat.

TASIKINESIA. Morbid inclination to get up and walk.

TEGMENTAL REACTION. *See* page 41.

TEONANACATL. *See* page 128.

TETRABENAZINE. *See* page 33.

TETRAHYDROCANNABINOL. *See* page 151.

TETRAHYDROHARMANE. *See* page 139.

TETRAHYDROHARMINE. *See* page 138.

TETRAHYDRONAPHTYLAMINE. *See* page 121.

THALAMOCORTICAL. Nervous pathways between the thalamus and the cortex.

THIOPROPERAZINE. *See* page 9.

THIORIDAZINE. *See* page 9.

THROMBOSIS. Formation of a clot in a blood vessel.

THYROXIN. Thyroid hormone.

TIOPENTAL. A BARBITURATE derivative.

TONIC-CLONIC. *See* CONVULSION.

TORTICOLLIS. Contracted state of the cervical muscles, leading to an unnatural position of the head.

TRANQUILIZING. Calming.

TRANYLCYPROMINE. *See* page 62.

TREMORIGENIC. Inducing tremor.

TRICYCLIC ANTIDEPRESSANTS. *See* page 50.

TRIFLUPERIDOL. *See* page 37.

TRIHEXYPHENYDIL. *See* page 157.

3-4-5-TRIMETHOXYAMPHETAMINE. *See* page 108.

TRYPTAMINE. *See* pages 65, 129.

TYBAMATE. *See* page 76.

TYROSINE HYDROXYLASE. Enzyme that transforms tyrosine into DOPA (*see* page 33).

UML. *See* page 122.

VAGAL ATTACK. Condition in which the vagal or parasympathetic system dominates the general functions of the organism.

VASODILATATION. Usually refers to dilatation of arterioles, leading to increased blood supply.

VASOMOTOR. Affecting movements (dilatation or constriction) of blood vessels.

VASOPRESSOR. Increasing pressure (usually by constriction) of blood vessels.

VIROLA CALLOPHYLLOIDEA (MYRISTICACEAE). *See* page 133.

ZOXAZOLAMINE. *See* page 76.